IØ1Ø4124

On The Renal Diet:

Cooking and Eating Easy

Erica Amber Hatcher, RD, LDN

Copyright © 2018 Erica Amber Hatcher, RD, LDN

Published by CaryPress International. www.CaryPress.com

All rights reserved.

No part of this publication may be reproduced, stored in a retrieval system or

transmitted in any form or by any means, electronic, mechanical,

photocopying, recording or otherwise, without prior permission of the author.

TABLE OF CONTENTS

Desserts

Misc.

DEDICATION

To my mom for inspiring me with the relentless discipline and dedication to better her family's life.

Also, to my patients for the love and compassion which they bestow on me and each other and the inspiration that I derive from their courage to fight and eat their way to better health.

Renal Diet Restrictions

A renal diet is recommended for patients with renal disease or kidney failure. People with kidney failure require a specialty diet. Processing certain foods become more difficult as kidney function diminishes.

Wastes in the blood come from food and liquids that are consumed. People with kidney disease must adhere to a special diet to decrease the amount of waste in their blood. Following a kidney diet may also bolster kidney function and delay total kidney failure.

A kidney diet is low in sodium, phosphorous, and potassium and stresses the importance of consuming high-quality protein and limiting fluids. Some kidney diets may also call for limited potassium and calcium. Every person is different. Therefore, a dietician will work with each patient to come up with a kidney diet that is tailored to his or her needs.

Please discuss your specific and individual diet needs with your doctor or dietitian.

Sodium

Sodium is a mineral found in salt (sodium chloride), and it is widely used in food preparation. Salt is one of the most commonly used seasonings. Reducing salt/sodium in your diet is an important tool in controlling your kidney disease. It takes time to reduce the salt intake in your diet and the following recommendations can help.

- Do not use salt when cooking food.

- Do not put salt on food when you eat.

- Learn to read food labels. Avoid foods that have more than 300mg sodium per serving (or 600mg for a complete frozen dinner). Avoid foods that have salt listed in the first 4 or 5 items in the ingredient list.

- Do not eat ham, bacon, sausage, hot dogs, lunch meats, chicken tenders or nuggets, or regular canned soup. Only eat soups that have labels saying the sodium level is reduced – and then only eat 1 cup – not the whole can.

- Canned vegetables should say "no salt added".

- Do not use flavored salts such as garlic salt, onion salt or "seasoned" salt. Also, avoid kosher or sea salt.

- Be sure to look for lower salt or "no salt added" options for your favorite foods such as peanut butter or box mixes.

- Do not purchase refrigerated or frozen meats that are packaged "in a solution"; or pre-seasoned/flavored. These items are usually chicken breasts, pork chops, pork tenderloin, steaks, or burgers.

Potassium

Potassium is a mineral involved in how muscles work. When kidneys do not function properly, potassium builds up in the blood. This can cause changes in how the heart beats and possibly lead to a heart attack. Potassium is found primarily in fruits, vegetables, milk, and meats. You will need to avoid certain ones and limit the amount of others.

Potassium-rich foods to avoid:

- Melons such as cantaloupe and honeydew (watermelon is okay)

- Bananas

- Oranges and orange juice

- Grapefruit juice

- Prune juice

- Tomatoes, tomato sauce, tomato juice

- Dried beans – all kinds

- Pumpkin

- Winter squash

- Cooked greens, spinach, kale, collards, Swiss Chard

Other foods to avoid include bran cereals, granola, "salt substitute" or "lite" salt, and molasses. Potatoes and sweet potatoes need special handling to allow you to eat them in SMALL amounts. Peel them, cut them in small slices or cubes and soak them for several hours in a large amount of water. When you are ready to cook them, pour the soaking water off and use a large amount of water in the pan. Drain this water before you prepare them to eat.

Be sure to eat a wide variety of fruits and vegetables every day to avoid getting too much potassium.

Phosphorus

Phosphorus is another mineral that can build up in your blood when your kidneys do not function. When this happens, calcium can be pulled from your bones and can collect in your skin or blood vessels. Bone disease can then become a problem, making a bone break more likely. The following should be taken into consideration to prevent the build-up of phosphorus in your blood.

- Dairy foods are the major source of phosphorus in the diet, so limit milk to 1 cup per day. If you use yogurt or cheese instead of liquid milk – only one container or 1 ounce a day!

- Some vegetables also contain phosphorus. Limit these to 1 cup per week: dried beans, greens, broccoli, mushrooms, and Brussels sprouts.

- Certain cereals need to be limited to 1 serving a week: bran, wheat cereals, oatmeal, and granola.

- White bread is better than whole grain breads or crackers.

- Soft drinks contain phosphorus so only drink clear ones, such as ginger ale. Do not drink Mountain Dew® (any kind), colas, root beers, Dr. Pepper® (any kind). Also, avoid Hawaiian Punch®, Fruitworks®, Cool® iced tea, and Aquafina® tangerine pineapple.

- Beer also has phosphorus – avoid all kinds.

Meat/Protein

People on dialysis need to eat more protein. Protein can help maintain blood protein levels and improve health. Eat a high protein food (meat, fish, poultry, fresh pork, or eggs) at every meal, or about 8-10 ounces of high protein foods everyday.

3 ounce = the size of a deck of cards, a medium pork chop, a 1/4 pound precooked weight hamburger patty, ½ chicken breast, a medium fish fillet.

1 ounce = 1 egg or 1/4 cup egg, 1/4 cup tuna, 1/4 cup ricotta cheese, 1 slice of low sodium lunchmeat.

Note: Even though peanut butter, nuts, seeds, dried beans, peas, and lentils have protein, these foods are generally not recommended because they are high in both potassium and phosphorus.

Grains/Cereals/Bread

Unless you need to limit your calorie intake for weight loss and/or manage carbohydrate intake for blood sugar control, you may eat as you desire from this food group. Grains, cereals, and breads are a good source of calories. Most people need 6 -11 servings from this group each day.

Amounts equal to one serving:

- 1 slice of bread (white, rye, or sourdough)
- ½ English muffin
- ½ bagel
- ½ hamburger bun
- ½ hot dog bun
- 1 6-inch tortilla
- ½ cup cooked pasta
- ½ cup cooked white rice
- ½ cup cooked cereal (like Cream of Wheat®)
- 1 cup cold cereal (like corn flakes or crispy rice)
- 4 unsalted crackers
- 1½ cups unsalted popcorn
- 10 vanilla wafers

Avoid "whole grain" and "high fiber" foods (like whole wheat bread, bran cereal and brown rice) to help you limit your intake of phosphorus. By limiting dairy–based foods you protect your bones and blood vessels.

Milk/Yogurt/Cheese

Limit your intake of milk, yogurt, and cheese to ½-cup milk or ½-cup yogurt or 1-ounce cheese per day. Most dairy foods are very high in phosphorus.

The phosphorus content is the same for all types of milk – skim, low fat, and whole! If you do eat any high-phosphorus foods, take a phosphate binder with that meal.

Dairy foods "low" in phosphorus:
(ask your dietitian about the serving size that is right for you)

- Butter and tub margarine

- Cream cheese

- Heavy cream

- Ricotta cheese

- Brie cheese

- Non-dairy whipped topping

- Sherbet

If you have or are at risk for heart disease, some of the high fat foods listed above may not be good choices for you.

Certain brands of non-dairy creams and "milk" (such as rice milk) are low in phosphorus and potassium. Ask your dietitian for details.

Fruit/Juice

All fruits have some potassium, but certain fruits have more than others and should be limited or totally avoided. Limiting potassium protects your heart.

Limit or avoid:

- Oranges and orange juice
- Raisins and dried fruit

- Kiwis
- Bananas

- Nectarines
- Melons (cantaloupe and honeydew)

- Prunes and prune juice

Always AVOID star fruit (carambola).

Eat 2-3 servings of low potassium fruits each day.
One serving = ½-cup or 1 small fruit or 4 ounces of juice.

Choose:

- Apple (1)
- Pear, fresh or canned, drained (1 half)

- Berries (½ cup)

- Cherries (10)

- Fruit cocktail, drained (½ cup)

- Grapes (15)

- Peach (1 small fresh or canned, drained)

- Pineapple (1/2 cup canned, drained)

- Plums (1-2)

- Tangerine (1)

- Watermelon (1 small wedge)

Drinks:

- Apple cider

- Cranberry juice cocktail

- Grape juice

- Lemonade

Vegetables/Salads

All vegetables have some potassium, but certain vegetables have more than others and should be limited or totally avoided. Limiting potassium intake protects your heart.

Eat 2-3 servings of low-potassium vegetables each day. One serving = 1/2 cup.

Choose:

- Broccoli (raw or cooked from frozen)

- Cabbage

- Carrots

- Cauliflower

- Celery

- Cucumber

- Eggplant

- Garlic

- Green and wax beans ("string beans")

- Lettuce-all types (1 cup)

- Onion

- Peppers-all types and colors

- Radishes

- Watercress

- Zucchini and yellow squash

Limit or avoid:

- Potatoes (including French Fries, potato chips and sweet potatoes)

- Avocado

- Beets

- Tomatoes and tomato sauce
- Winter squash
- Pumpkin
- Asparagus (cooked)
- Beet greens
- Cooked spinach
- Parsnips and rutabaga

Dessert

Depending on your calorie needs, your dietitian may recommend high-calorie deserts. Pies, cookies, sherbet, and cakes are good choices (but limit dairy-based desserts and those made with chocolate, nuts, and bananas). If you are a diabetic, discuss low carbohydrate dessert choices with your dietitian.

Sample Menu:

Breakfast:

Cranberry Juice, 4 ounces
Eggs (2) or ½-cup egg substitute
Toasted white bread, 2 slices, with Butter or tub margarine or fruit spread
Coffee, 6 ounces

Lunch:

Tuna salad sandwich made with 3 ounces tuna on a hard roll with lettuce and mayonnaise.
(Other good choices for sandwiches include egg and chicken salad, lean roast beef, low salt ham and turkey breast.)
Coleslaw, 1/2 cup
Pretzels, 15
Canned and drained peaches, 1/2 cup
Ginger ale, 8 ounces

(Cola drinks are high in phosphorus. Choose ginger ale or lemon-lime beverages instead.)

Dinner:

Hamburger patty, 4 ounces on a bun with 1-2 teaspoons ketchup
Salad (1 cup): lettuce, cucumber, radishes, peppers, with olive oil and vinegar dressing
Lemonade, 8 ounces

Aim for at least 2-3 "fish" meals each week. Many fish are rich in heart-healthy "omega-3" fats. Tuna and salmon (rinsed or canned without salt) and shellfish are excellent heart healthy protein choices.

Snack/Dessert

Milk, 4 ounces
Slice of apple pie, 1/8 slice

This meal plan provides 2150 Calories, 91 grams protein, 2300 mg sodium, 1800 mg (46 mEq) potassium, 950 mg phosphorus. 38 ounces of oral fluid.

Organic vs. Inorganic

The word "organic" refers to the way farmers grow and process agricultural products, such as fruits, vegetables, grains, dairy products and meat. Organic farming practices are designed to encourage soil and water conservation and reduce pollution.

Farmers who grow organic produce do not use conventional methods to fertilize and control weeds. Examples of organic farming practices include using natural fertilizers to feed soil and plants, and using crop rotation or mulch to manage weeds.

100 percent organic. To use this phrase, products must be either completely organic or made of all organic ingredients.

Organic. Products must be at least 95 percent organic to use this term.

Organic can be pricey, I know when you are on a limited budget you may hesitate to purchase organic food items.

Canned goods are okay to purchase. Simply reduce some of the sodium intake by rinsing the goods inside the can with water and/or discard the juices from within.

For the recipes, try to use as many fresh ingredients as possible. Feel free to tweak recipes to suit your palate.

Breakfast & Brunch

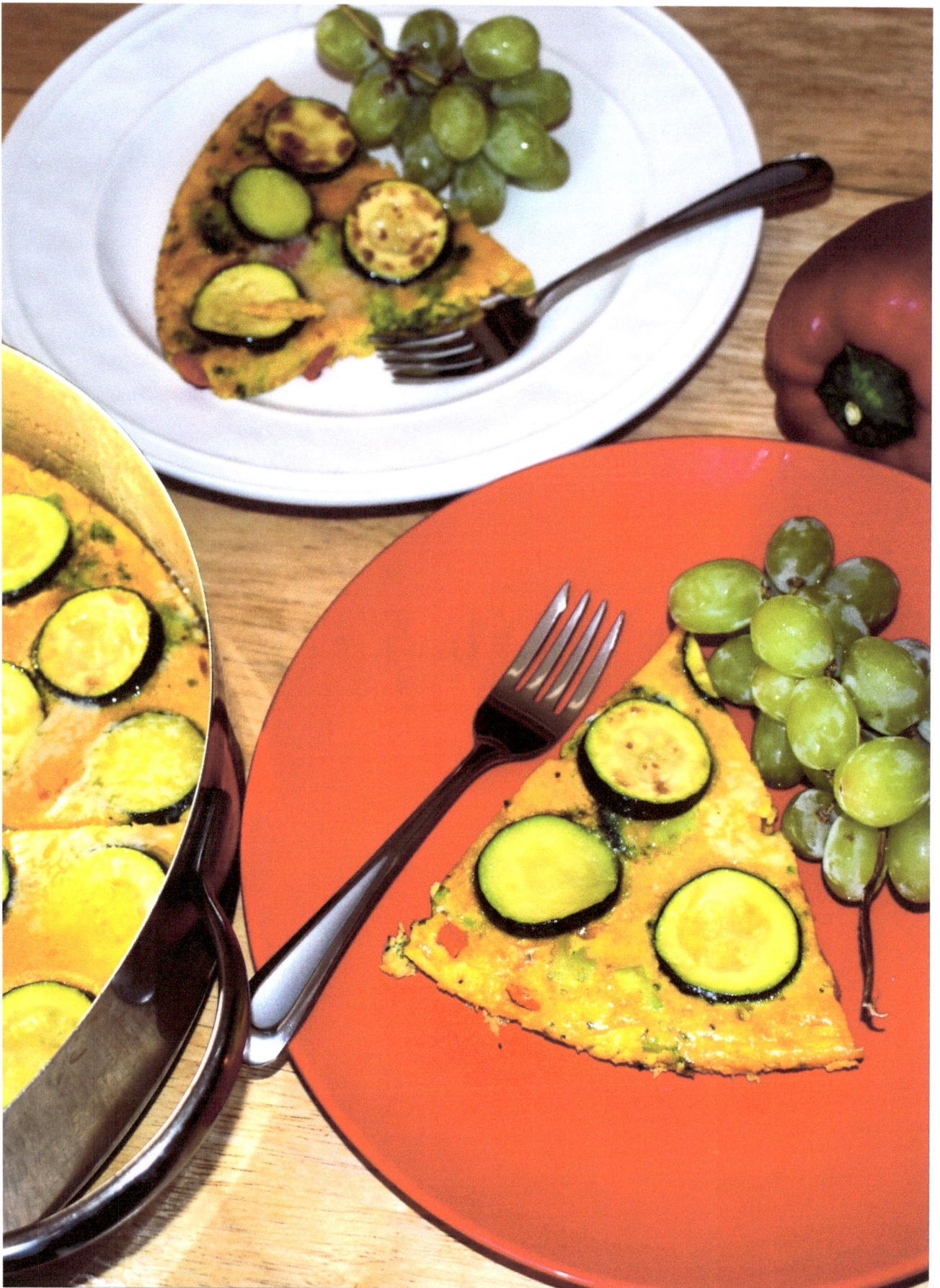

Breakfast Frittata

Ingredients

- 4 eggs (lightly beaten)

- 1 scallion (diced)

- 1 red pepper (diced)

- 1/4 cup fresh broccoli (chopped small)

- 1 zucchini (sliced, then diced small)

- 1/4 tsp salt

- 1 tsp cayenne pepper

- 2 tsp grated Parmesan cheese

- PAM® cooking spray

Instructions

1. Preheat oven to 375 degrees

2. Spray non-stick small oven-proof pan with PAM® cooking spray (coat well).

3. Add scallions, red pepper, broccoli, and zucchini.

4. Sauté on low heat for approximately 8 minutes or until vegetables become tender dry.

5. In a bowl lightly beat eggs and add salt and cayenne pepper.

6. Add eggs to the sauté pan.

7. Sprinkle Parmesan cheese on top of mixture in the pan.

8. Place in oven and bake for approximately 20 minutes.

Nutrition Facts

Servings: 4

Amount per serving

Calories	130

	% Daily Value*
Total Fat 7.7g	10%
Saturated Fat 3.4g	17%
Cholesterol 174mg	58%
Sodium 347mg	15%
Total Carbohydrate 5.6g	2%
Dietary Fiber 1.3g	5%
Total Sugars 2.9g	
Protein 11.2g	
Vitamin D 15mcg	77%
Calcium 164mg	13%
Iron 1mg	7%
Potassium 281mg	6%

*The % Daily Value (DV) tells you how much a nutrient in a food serving contributes to a daily diet. 2,000 calorie a day is used for general nutrition advice.

Chicken, Broccoli Quiche

Ingredients

- 1 frozen 10 inch pie crust

- 2 tablespoons unsalted butter

- 1/2 cup chopped onion

- 2 garlic cloves minced

- 1 cup cooked broccoli diced

- 1 cup cooked chicken diced

- 1/4 teaspoon salt

- 1/4 teaspoon pepper

- 5 eggs

- 1 cup rice milk

- 1 cup freshly grated cheddar cheese

- 1 tablespoon flour

Instructions

1. Preheat oven to 350 degrees. Using a fork, poke holes around the sides of the pie crust. Sprinkle flour on the bottom of the pie crust.

2. Set the pie in the oven for 10 minutes, and then remove.

3. Heat the butter in a large skillet over medium-high heat. Add the onion and cook, stirring, until lightly browned. Add the broccoli, chicken, salt, and pepper and stir to combine.

4. In a bowl, whisk together the eggs and milk. Add the vegetable mixture and cheese and mix well. Pour the mixture into the crust and bake for 15 minutes.

5. Reduce the oven temperature to 325 degrees and bake until just set around the edges but slightly loose in the center, about 30 to 40 minutes. Let the filling set and cool before serving.

Nutrition Facts

Servings: 6

Amount per serving

Calories 224

% Daily Value*

Total Fat 13.5g	17%
Saturated Fat 6.3g	31%
Cholesterol 178mg	59%
Sodium 381mg	17%
Total Carbohydrate 9.7g	4%
Dietary Fiber 0.7g	3%
Total Sugars 1.1g	
Protein 17g	
Vitamin D 15mcg	77%
Calcium 306mg	24%
Iron 1mg	7%
Potassium 177mg	4%

*The % Daily Value (DV) tells you how much a nutrient in a food serving contributes to a daily diet. 2,000 calorie a day is used for general nutrition advice.

Homemade Drop Biscuits

Ingredients

- 2 cups all purpose flour

- 1 tablespoon baking powder

- 2 teaspoons white sugar

- 1/2 teaspoon cream of tartar

- 1/4 teaspoon salt

- 1/2 cup melted butter

- 1 cup rice milk

Instructions

1. Preheat oven to 450 degrees.

2. In a large bowl, combine flour, baking powder, sugar, cream of tartar and salt. Stir in butter and milk just until moistened. Drop batter on a lightly greased cookie sheet by the tablespoon.

3. Bake in preheated oven until golden on the edges, about 8 to 12 minutes. Serve warm.

Nutrition Facts

Servings: 8

Amount per serving

Calories	237

	% Daily Value*
Total Fat 12.1g	15%
Saturated Fat 7.4g	37%
Cholesterol 31mg	10%
Sodium 169mg	7%
Total Carbohydrate 29g	11%
Dietary Fiber 0.9g	3%
Total Sugars 1.1g	
Protein 3.4g	
Vitamin D 8mcg	40%
Calcium 92mg	7%
Iron 2mg	9%
Potassium 267mg	6%

*The % Daily Value (DV) tells you how much a nutrient in a food serving contributes to a daily diet. 2,000 calorie a day is used for general nutrition advice.

Blueberry Breakfast Smoothie

Ingredients

- 1 cup fresh blueberries

- 1/2 cup Greek yogurt

- 1/4 cup cranberry juice

- 1 tablespoon agave nectar

- 1/4 teaspoon vanilla extract

- 1 pinch ground cinnamon, or to taste

- 3 ice cubes

Instructions

1. Blend blueberries, yogurt, cranberry juice, agave nectar, vanilla extract, and cinnamon together in a blender on low speed for 30 seconds; increase speed to high and blend until smooth, about 2 minutes.

2. Add ice and blend on high until smooth, about 1 minute more.

Nutrition Facts

Servings: 4

Amount per serving

Calories	**105**

% Daily Value*

Total Fat 0.6g	1%
Saturated Fat 0.4g	2%
Cholesterol 1mg	0%
Sodium 10mg	0%
Total Carbohydrate 23.3g	8%
Dietary Fiber 2.4g	9%
Total Sugars 19.9g	
Protein 2.8g	
Vitamin D 0mcg	0%
Calcium 33mg	3%
Iron 1mg	3%
Potassium 78mg	2%

*The % Daily Value (DV) tells you how much a nutrient in a food serving contributes to a daily diet. 2,000 calorie a day is used for general nutrition advice.

Classic Pancakes

Ingredients

- 1-1/2 cups all-purpose flour

- 3-1/2 teaspoons baking powder

- 1/4 teaspoon salt

- 1 tablespoon white sugar

- 1-1/4 non-dairy milk (or rice milk)

- 1 egg

- 3 tablespoons butter, melted

Instructions

1. In a large bowl, sift together the flour, baking powder, salt and sugar. Make a well in the center and pour in the milk, egg and melted butter; mix until smooth.

2. Heat a lightly oiled griddle or frying pan over medium high heat. Pour or scoop the batter onto the griddle, using approximately 1/4 cup for each pancake. Brown on both sides and serve hot.

Nutrition Facts

Servings: 4

Amount per serving

Calories	316

% Daily Value*

Total Fat 10.8g	14%
Saturated Fat 5.9g	30%
Cholesterol 64mg	21%
Sodium 256mg	11%
Total Carbohydrate 48.7g	18%
Dietary Fiber 1.4g	5%
Total Sugars 3.2g	
Protein 6.4g	
Vitamin D 10mcg	49%
Calcium 211mg	16%
Iron 3mg	16%
Potassium 531mg	11%

*The % Daily Value (DV) tells you how much a nutrient in a food serving contributes to a daily diet. 2,000 calorie a day is used for general nutrition advice.

Breakfast Egg Muffin Cups

Ingredients

- 2 cups spinach, chopped

- 1 large roma tomato, seeds removed and diced

- 1/2 green onion diced

- 1 jalapeno, seeded and diced

- 12 eggs

- 1/4 cup unsweetened non-dairy milk (or any milk)

- 1/2 teaspoon salt

- 1 tsp ground black pepper

Instructions

1. Preheat oven to 350 degrees. Spray a muffin tin with nonstick cooking spray.

2. Divide spinach, tomatoes, green onion, and jalapeño evenly between 12 muffins in the tin.

Nutrition Facts

Servings: 6

Amount per serving

Calories	**148**
	% Daily Value*
Total Fat 9.1g	**12%**
Saturated Fat 2.8g	**14%**
Cholesterol 327mg	**109%**
Sodium 334mg	**15%**
Total Carbohydrate 5.5g	**2%**
Dietary Fiber 1.1g	**4%**
Total Sugars 2.5g	
Protein 12.1g	
Vitamin D 31mcg	154%
Calcium 60mg	5%
Iron 3mg	19%
Potassium 326mg	7%

*The % Daily Value (DV) tells you how much a nutrient in a food serving contributes to a daily diet. 2,000 calorie a day is used for general nutrition advice.

3. In a large bowl whisk together eggs, milk, salt and pepper until well combined.

4. Fill each muffin tin about 3/4 full with egg mixture, pouring over the veggies already in each tin. Bake for 25-30 minutes until eggs are set and puff up in the tin. Let muffins cool for a few minutes, then run a butter knife around the edges of each cup and remove. Serves 6 (2 egg cups each).

Snacks

Seasoned Snack Pretzels

Ingredients

- 32 ounces unsalted pretzels (two 16-oz bags)

- 1 cup canola oil

- 2 tablespoons Hidden Valley®

    Ranch Salad Dressing and Seasoning mix

- 3 teaspoons garlic powder

Instructions

1. Preheat oven to 175° F.

2. Spread the pretzels out on two large cookie sheets, so that pretzels lay flat.

3. Mix the garlic powder and dill together. Set aside half of the seasonings. To the other half, add the dry salad dressing mix and 3/4 cup canola oil. Pour evenly over the pretzels, making sure pretzels are evenly coated.

4. Bake for 1 hour, flipping the pretzels every 15 minutes.

5. Remove the pretzels from the oven. Let the pretzels cool, then toss with remaining garlic powder, and oil.

Nutrition Facts	
Servings: 16	
Amount per serving	
Calories	**323**
	% Daily Value*
Total Fat 13.6g	17%
Saturated Fat 1g	5%
Cholesterol 0mg	0%
Sodium 213mg	9%
Total Carbohydrate 44.6g	16%
Dietary Fiber 2g	7%
Total Sugars 0.1g	
Protein 6.1g	
Vitamin D 0mcg	0%
Calcium 0mg	0%
Iron 1mg	4%
Potassium 6mg	0%

The % Daily Value (DV) tells you how much a nutrient in a food serving contributes to a daily diet. 2,000 calorie a day is used for general nutrition advice.

Turkey Bacon Deviled Eggs

Ingredients

- 12 eggs

- 1/2 cup light mayonnaise

- 4 slices turkey bacon

- 2 tablespoons finely shredded sharp cheddar cheese

- 1 tablespoon mustard

- 1 tbsp relish

Instructions

1. Place eggs in a saucepan, and cover with cold water. Bring water to a boil and immediately remove from heat. Cover, and let eggs stand in hot water for 10 to 12 minutes. Remove from hot water, and cool. To cool more quickly, rinse eggs under cold running water.

2. Meanwhile, place bacon in a large, deep skillet. Cook over medium-high heat until evenly brown. Alternatively, wrap bacon in paper towels and cook in the microwave for about 1 minute per slice. Crumble and set aside.

3. Peel the hard-cooked eggs, and cut in half lengthwise. Remove yolks to a small bowl. Mash egg yolks with mayonnaise, crumbled turkey bacon and cheese. Stir in mustard. Fill egg white halves with the yolk mixture and refrigerate until serving.

Nutrition Facts

Servings: 12

Amount per serving

Calories 119

	% Daily Value*
Total Fat 8.5g	11%
Saturated Fat 2.1g	11%
Cholesterol 171mg	57%
Sodium 189mg	8%
Total Carbohydrate 3.5g	1%
Dietary Fiber 0.2g	1%
Total Sugars 1.4g	
Protein 7.2g	
Vitamin D 16mcg	78%
Calcium 38mg	3%
Iron 1mg	5%
Potassium 68mg	1%

*The % Daily Value (DV) tells you how much a nutrient in a food serving contributes to a daily diet. 2,000 calorie a day is used for general nutrition advice.

Hot Crab Dip

Ingredients

- 8 ounces cream cheese

- 4 ounces sour cream

- 2 tablespoon onion minced

- 1 teaspoon lemon juice

- 2 teaspoons Worcestershire sauce

- 1 teaspoon black pepper

- 1 teaspoon hot sauce

- 1 teaspoon garlic powder

- 12 ounces jumbo lump crab meat

Instructions

1. Preheat the oven to 375 degrees. Set cream cheese out to soften. Finely mince the onion.

2. Place softened cream cheese in a bowl.

3. Add the onion, sour cream, lemon juice, Worcestershire sauce, garlic powder, black pepper and hot sauce. Mix well.

4. Add the jumbo lump crab meat and stir until blended.

5. Place mixture into an oven-safe dish. Bake uncovered for 15-20 minutes or until hot and bubbly.

Nutrition Facts

Servings: 4

Amount per serving

Calories	**343**

	% Daily Value*
Total Fat 27.3g	35%
Saturated Fat 16.2g	81%
Cholesterol 120mg	40%
Sodium 775mg	34%
Total Carbohydrate 6.1g	2%
Dietary Fiber 0.3g	1%
Total Sugars 1.1g	
Protein 16.1g	
Vitamin D 0mcg	0%
Calcium 386mg	30%
Iron 2mg	11%
Potassium 133mg	3%

*The % Daily Value (DV) tells you how much a nutrient in a food serving contributes to a daily diet. 2,000 calorie a day is used for general nutrition advice.

Soups & Salads

Spring Fruit Salad

Ingredients

- 2/3 cup fresh cranberry juice
- 1/3 cup fresh lemon juice
- 1/3 cup packed brown sugar
- 1/2 teaspoon grated orange zest
- 1/2 teaspoon grated lemon zest
- 1 teaspoon vanilla extract
- 2 cups cubed fresh pineapple
- 2 cups strawberries, hulled and sliced
- 3 kiwi fruit, peeled and sliced
- 1 banana, sliced
- 2 mandarin oranges, peeled and sectioned
- 1-1/2 cup seedless grapes
- 2 cups blueberries

Nutrition Facts

Servings: 6

Amount per serving

Calories	**185**

	% Daily Value*
Total Fat 0.8g	1%
Saturated Fat 0.2g	1%
Cholesterol 0mg	0%
Sodium 10mg	0%
Total Carbohydrate 45.3g	16%
Dietary Fiber 5.6g	20%
Total Sugars 34.5g	
Protein 2.2g	
Vitamin D 0mcg	0%
Calcium 47mg	4%
Iron 2mg	8%
Potassium 509mg	11%

*The % Daily Value (DV) tells you how much a nutrient in a food serving contributes to a daily diet. 2,000 calorie a day is used for general nutrition advice.

Instructions

1. Bring cranberry juice, lemon juice, brown sugar, orange zest, and lemon zest to a boil in a saucepan over medium-high heat. Reduce heat to medium-low, and simmer until slightly thickened, about 5 minutes. Remove from heat, and stir in vanilla extract. Set aside to cool.

2. Layer the fruit in a large, clear glass bowl in this order: pineapple, strawberries, kiwi fruit, banana, mandarin oranges, grapes, and blueberries. Pour the cooled sauce over the fruit. Cover and refrigerate for 4 hours before serving.

Coleslaw

Ingredients

- 2 cups cabbage

- 1/4 cup carrots

- 2 tablespoons green bell peppers diced

- 2 tablespoons yellow pepper diced

- 1/4 cup onion diced

- 1/4 cup light mayonnaise

- 2 tablespoons vinegar

- 1/4 tablespoon sugar

- 1/2 teaspoon black pepper

- 1/4 teaspoon celery seed

Nutrition Facts

Servings: 4

Amount per serving

Calories 103

% Daily Value*

Total Fat 5.2g	7%
Saturated Fat 0.7g	4%
Cholesterol 4mg	1%
Sodium 119mg	5%
Total Carbohydrate 14.1g	5%
Dietary Fiber 2.3g	8%
Total Sugars 6.5g	
Protein 1.6g	
Vitamin D 0mcg	0%
Calcium 32mg	2%
Iron 1mg	4%
Potassium 271mg	6%

*The % Daily Value (DV) tells you how much a nutrient in a food serving contributes to a daily diet. 2,000 calorie a day is used for general nutrition advice.

Instructions

1. Combine all vegetables together.

2. In small bowl blend mayonnaise, vinegar, sugar and seasonings and pour over vegetables. Mix.

Chopped Salad

Ingredients

- 1/2 cup finely chopped red onions

- 1/4 cup water

- 1/2 cup red wine vinegar

- 1/4 teaspoons kosher salt, plus additional as needed

- 2 teaspoon coarsely ground fresh black pepper, plus additional as needed

- 1/2 to 1 cup extra virgin olive oil

- 1 large head iceberg lettuce, cut into 1/2-inch pieces, 6 to 8 cups

- 1 cup finely chopped carrots

- 1/2 cup chopped green onions

- 1 cucumber, peeled and cut into 1/2-inch pieces

- 1/4 cup flat-leaf parsley leaves

- 1/4 cup coarsely chopped dill, large stems removed

Nutrition Facts

Servings: 4

Amount per serving

Calories 285

% Daily Value*

Total Fat 25.7g	33%
Saturated Fat 3.6g	18%
Cholesterol 0mg	0%
Sodium 186mg	8%
Total Carbohydrate 14.6g	5%
Dietary Fiber 3.3g	12%
Total Sugars 5.6g	
Protein 2.2g	
Vitamin D 0mcg	0%
Calcium 52mg	4%
Iron 6mg	35%
Potassium 585mg	12%

*The % Daily Value (DV) tells you how much a nutrient in a food serving contributes to a daily diet. 2,000 calorie a day is used for general nutrition advice.

Instructions

1. In a small bowl, combine the onions, water, vinegar, salt, and pepper. Let sit at room temperature for 10 minutes to allow the flavors to develop.

2. Add 1/2 cup of the olive oil to the vinegar mixture. Add additional to taste.

3. In a large bowl, combine the lettuce, cucumber, carrots, green onion, and herbs. Toss with enough dressing to coat, and season to taste with additional salt and pepper. Serve any remaining dressing on the side.

Erica Amber Hatcher, RD, LDN

Corn and Kale Salad

Ingredients

- 4 ears sweet corn, husked

- 1 bunch kale – stems removed and discarded, leaves torn into bite-size pieces

- 2 cups chopped iceberg lettuce

- 1 large red bell pepper, chopped

- 1/4 cup pineapple juice

- 1/4 cup olive oil

- 2 tablespoons salsa

- 2 teaspoons Mrs. Dash®, or to taste

- 1 teaspoon garlic powder

- 1 teaspoon onion powder

- 1/4 tsp salt

- 1 tsp black pepper

Nutrition Facts

Servings: 4

Amount per serving

Calories 278

% Daily Value*

Total Fat 14.6g	19%
Saturated Fat 2.1g	11%
Cholesterol 0mg	0%
Sodium 229mg	10%
Total Carbohydrate 37.7g	14%
Dietary Fiber 5.4g	19%
Total Sugars 9g	
Protein 6.4g	
Vitamin D 0mcg	0%
Calcium 35mg	3%
Iron 5mg	30%
Potassium 662mg	14%

*The % Daily Value (DV) tells you how much a nutrient in a food serving contributes to a daily diet. 2,000 calorie a day is used for general nutrition advice.

Instructions

1. Bring a large pot of water to a boil. Add corn to boiling water and turn off heat. Let corn soak in hot water for 5 minutes. Remove the corn, reserving the cooking water in the pot. Set corn aside to cool before slicing kernels from the cobs into a mixing bowl.

2. Return the pot of water to a boil; add kale and 1 teaspoon salt. Boil kale until bright green and tender, about 3- 5 minutes; drain and set kale aside to cool. Once cool enough to handle, squeeze as much liquid from the kale as you can. Combine kale, iceberg lettuce and corn kernels to a large bowl.

3. Stir red bell pepper, pineapple juice, olive oil, salsa, Mrs. Dash® seasoning, garlic powder, and onion powder into the corn, kale, and iceberg bowl.

Homemade Hearty Vegetable Soup

Ingredients

- 1 cup fresh green beans

- 3/4 cup celery

- 1/4 cup onion

- 1 small white potato peeled

- 1/2 cup carrots

- 1 medium Roma tomato

- 2 tablespoons olive oil

- 1 cup frozen corn

- 4 cups low-sodium vegetable broth

- 1 teaspoon dried parsley leaves

- 1 teaspoon garlic powder

- 1/4 teaspoon salt

Nutrition Facts	
Servings: 4	
Amount per serving	
Calories	**160**
	% Daily Value*
Total Fat 7.6g	10%
Saturated Fat 1.1g	6%
Cholesterol 0mg	0%
Sodium 253mg	11%
Total Carbohydrate 20g	7%
Dietary Fiber 3.9g	14%
Total Sugars 3.9g	
Protein 5g	
Vitamin D 0mcg	0%
Calcium 28mg	2%
Iron 2mg	13%
Potassium 461mg	10%

*The % Daily Value (DV) tells you how much a nutrient in a food serving contributes to a daily diet. 2,000 calorie a day is used for general nutrition advice.

Instructions

1. Remove tips and strings from the green beans and cut into 2-inch pieces. Dice the celery, onion, carrots, potato and tomato.

2. In a large pot heat the olive oil and sauté the celery and onion until tender.

3. Add the remaining ingredients and bring to a boil. Reduce heat to a simmer and cook for 45 to 60 minutes.

Carrot Soup

Ingredients

- 3 pounds carrots, chopped

- 6 cups chicken stock

- 3 cloves garlic, chopped

- 2 tablespoons dried dill weed

- 1 tablespoon Butter

- 1/4 teaspoon salt

Instructions

1. In a medium sized stock pot, over high heat, combine the chicken stock, carrots, garlic, dill weed, salt and butter. Bring to a boil, reduce heat and simmer for 30 minutes or until carrots are soft.

2. In a blender, puree the soup, return to stock pot and simmer for an additional 30 to 45 minutes. Season with additional dill or garlic if needed.

Nutrition Facts

Servings: 6

Amount per serving

Calories 135

% Daily Value*

Total Fat 2g	3%
Saturated Fat 1.2g	6%
Cholesterol 5mg	2%
Sodium 399mg	17%
Total Carbohydrate 24.4g	9%
Dietary Fiber 5.8g	21%
Total Sugars 12.2g	
Protein 6.2g	
Vitamin D 1mcg	7%
Calcium 96mg	7%
Iron 2mg	9%
Potassium 1018mg	22%

The % Daily Value (DV) tells you how much a nutrient in a food serving contributes to a daily diet. 2,000 calorie a day is used for general nutrition advice.

Cream of Broccoli Soup

Ingredients

- 2 heads of fresh broccoli crowns

- 16 ounces of fresh vegetable broth

- 1 cup carrots diced

- 1 onion diced

- 1 cup water

- 1 medium potato, peeled and cubed

- 1/3 cup non-dairy creamer

- 4 garlic cloves, minced

- 1/4 teaspoon salt

- 1 teaspoon freshly ground black pepper

Instructions

1. Wash broccoli crowns and cut into quarters. Add broccoli, diced onions, potato, carrots, garlic, salt, pepper, vegetable broth and water to a large pot and boil. Boil until broccoli is tender. Use fork to see tenderness. Usually soft within 40 minutes. Turn fire off, and allow to get to warm temperature.

2. Next blend using a hand mixer, or soup mixer. (Note: you can use the hand mixer in the same pot) Blend on low until all ingredients are fully blended.

3. Once fully blended add 1/3 non-dairy creamer and blend on low for additional 2 minutes.

4. Reheat soup on low for about 5-10 minutes until desired temperature.

Nutrition Facts

Servings: 4

Amount per serving

Calories 102

% Daily Value*

Total Fat 0.9g	**1%**
Saturated Fat 0g	**0%**
Cholesterol 0mg	**0%**
Sodium 214mg	**9%**
Total Carbohydrate 21.2g	**8%**
Dietary Fiber 4.8g	**17%**
Total Sugars 4.5g	
Protein 4.2g	
Vitamin D 0mcg	0%
Calcium 73mg	6%
Iron 1mg	7%
Potassium 634mg	13%

*The % Daily Value (DV) tells you how much a nutrient in a food serving contributes to a daily diet. 2,000 calorie a day is used for general nutrition advice.

Lunch & Dinner

Baked Dijon Salmon

Ingredients

- 4 (3 oz salmon fillets)

- 1 tbsp unsalted butter (melted)

- 1-1/2 tablespoon Dijon mustard

- 1-1/2 tablespoon liquid honey

- 1/3 cup bread crumbs

- 4 tsp fresh parsley, chopped

- 1 tsp Mrs. Dash®

- 1 teaspoon black pepper

- 4 lemon wedges

Instructions

1. Preheat oven to 400 degrees.

2. Wash salmon fillets under cold running water.

3. In a small bowl stir together melted butter, mustard and honey (set aside).

4. In another bowl stir together the bread crumbs, and parsley.

5. Brush each salmon fillet lightly with honey mustard mixture, and sprinkle the tops of the fillets with the bread crumb mixture.

6. Bake the salmon fillets for 15-20 minutes in the preheated oven or until it flakes easily with a fork. Season with Mrs. Dash and pepper. Garnish with a lemon wedge

Nutrition Facts

Servings: 4

Amount per serving

Calories 121

% Daily Value*

Total Fat 5g	6%
Saturated Fat 2.1g	11%
Cholesterol 17mg	6%
Sodium 164mg	7%
Total Carbohydrate 14.4g	5%
Dietary Fiber 1g	4%
Total Sugars 7.3g	
Protein 18.3g	
Vitamin D 2mcg	10%
Calcium 35mg	3%
Iron 1mg	5%
Potassium 146mg	3%

*The % Daily Value (DV) tells you how much a nutrient in a food serving contributes to a daily diet. 2,000 calorie a day is used for general nutrition advice.

Erica Amber Hatcher, RD, LDN

Honey Garlic Chicken

Ingredients

- 4 chicken quarters (legs and thighs)

- 1/2 cup honey

- 2 tsp pepper

- 2 garlic cloves, minced

- 1/4 onion, finely chopped

- 3 tsp canola oil for frying

Instructions

1. Clean chicken thighs and legs under cold water, remove skin.

2. In a frying pan add canola oil, heat oil and add onion, garlic, pepper, chicken legs and thighs.

3. Cook for approximately 7-8 minutes on each side.

4. Remove chicken from heat and place in a casserole dish.

5. Add honey to the ingredients left in the frying pan and glaze the pan.

6. Pour mixture over chicken and cook for 40 minutes at 350? F.

Nutrition Facts

Servings: 4

Amount per serving

Calories	207

	% Daily Value*
Total Fat 6.1g	8%
Saturated Fat 1g	5%
Cholesterol 23mg	8%
Sodium 21mg	1%
Total Carbohydrate 36.7g	13%
Dietary Fiber 0.5g	2%
Total Sugars 35.1g	
Protein 20g	
Vitamin D 0mcg	0%
Calcium 15mg	1%
Iron 1mg	3%
Potassium 119mg	3%

*The % Daily Value (DV) tells you how much a nutrient in a food serving contributes to a daily diet. 2,000 calorie a day is used for general nutrition advice.

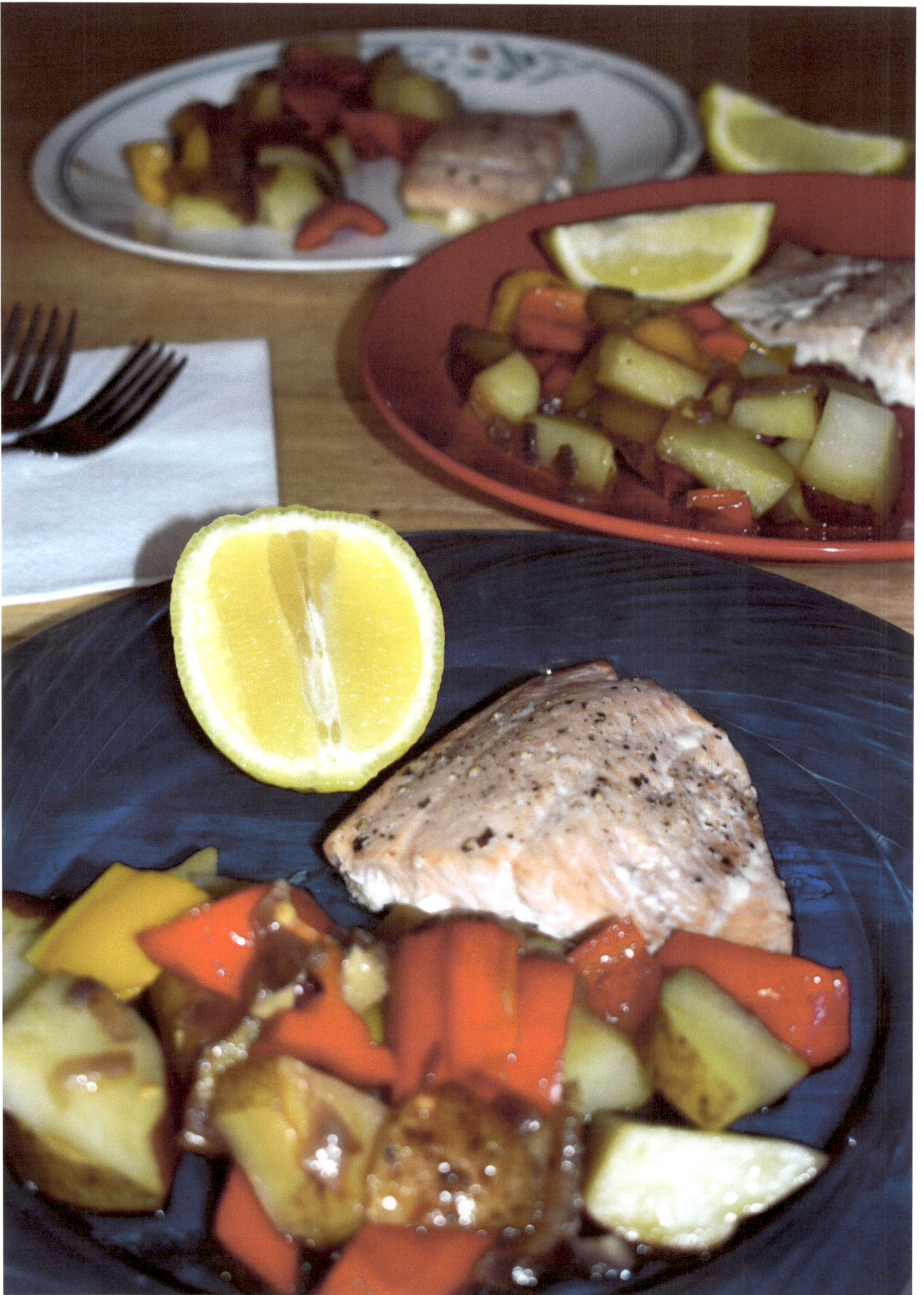

Lemon-wine Chilean Salmon

Ingredients

- 2 Chilean salmon fillets (12 oz)

- 1 tablespoon black pepper

- 2 tablespoon extra virgin olive oil

- 1 tablespoon unsalted butter

- 2 peppers sliced (one yellow/one red)

- 1/4 teaspoon kosher salt

- 1 small potato diced (Remember to peel, cut and soak for 4 hours)

- 1 onion sliced

- 2 tablespoon lemon juice

Instructions

1. Preheat oven to 325 degrees.

2. Place olive oil and butter in large pan. Saute' on medium temperature until butter and oil are fully melted.

3. Place salmon fillets in pan skin side down, cook for approximately 20 minutes.

4. Flip salmon fillets over to the other side, remove skin (skin should peel off easily).

5. Sprinkle kosher salt, wine, and pepper to the top of the fillets cook for approximately 10 minutes.

6. Add peppers, onions and potatoes to the pan beside the salmon.

7. Pour the lemon juice on top of the fillets. Add items to a casserole dish

8. Bake for approximately 30 minutes.

Nutrition Facts

Servings: 4

Amount per serving

Calories   155

	% Daily Value*
Total Fat 10.2g	13%
Saturated Fat 2.9g	15%
Cholesterol 8mg	3%
Sodium 175mg	8%
Total Carbohydrate 15.7g	6%
Dietary Fiber 2.8g	10%
Total Sugars 4.7g	
Protein 18.3g	
Vitamin D 2mcg	10%
Calcium 25mg	2%
Iron 1mg	6%
Potassium 362mg	8%

*The % Daily Value (DV) tells you how much a nutrient in a food serving contributes to a daily diet. 2,000 calorie a day is used for general nutrition advice.

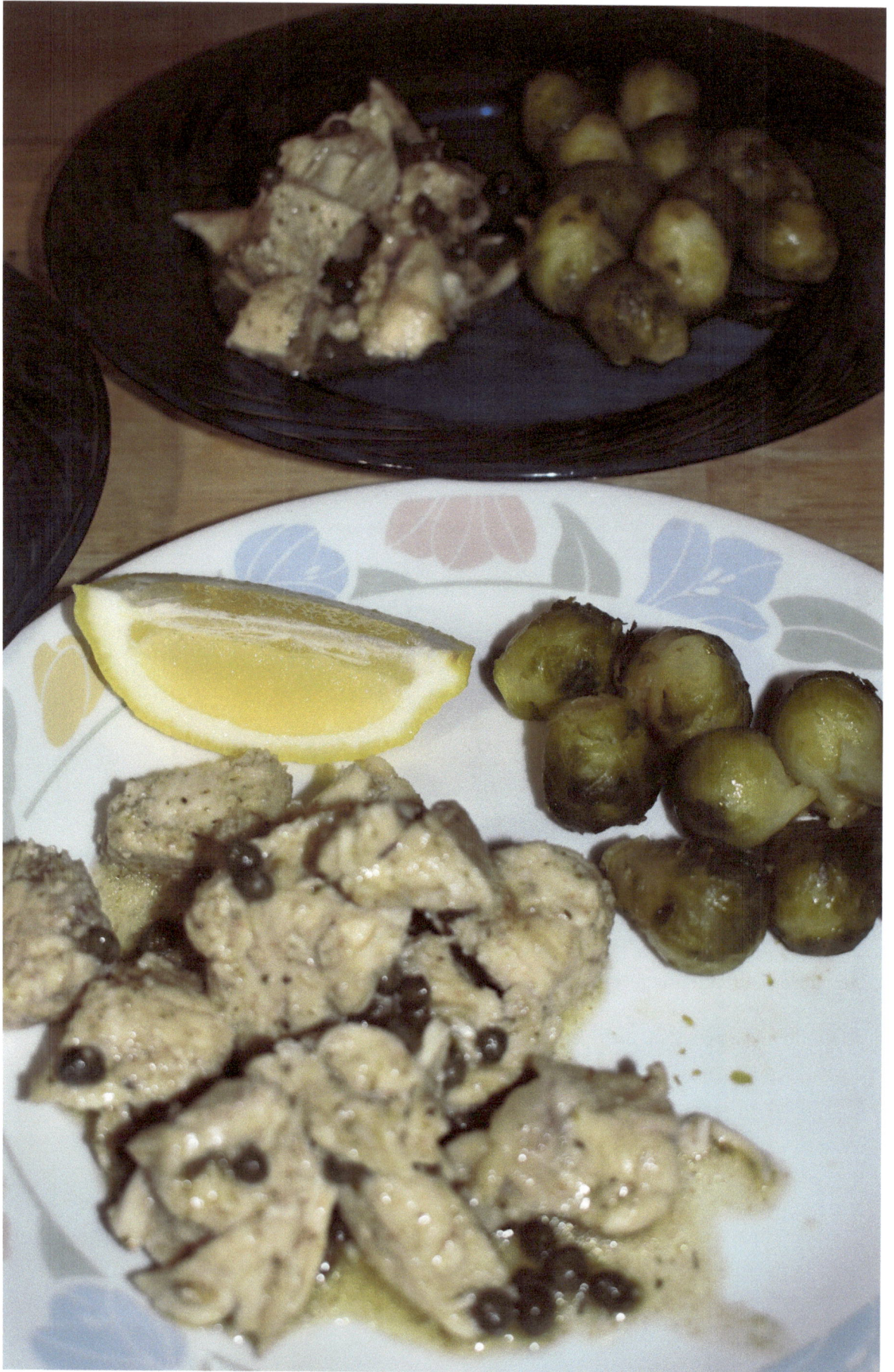

Rosemary Chicken with Caper Sauce

Ingredients

- 1 pound of boneless skinless chicken breasts

- 1 teaspoon black pepper

- 2 teaspoon capers (drained)

- 1 teaspoon lemon juice

- 2 tbsp flour

- 3 tablespoon red cooking wine

- 1 tablespoon extra virgin olive oil

- 2 tablespoon fresh rosemary or 2 stems of fresh rosemary

- 1/2 cup water

Instructions

1. Wash chicken breasts under cold water. Cut chicken breasts in cubes.

2. In a large sauce pan add oil, heat for 2-3 minutes on medium temperature.

3. Add chicken breasts to oil; stir the chicken so that all the chicken is covered with some of the oil.

4. Add in the rosemary, lemon juice, pepper and sauté for around 7 minutes.

5. Remove the chicken cubes from the sauce pan; leave the chicken stock in the pan.

6. In a small cup add water, and flour and blend until it is smooth. Add to the chicken stock.

7. Next add the red wine and let simmer. Once the sauce comes to a rapid simmer. Add the drained capers.

8. As the sauce starts to thicken, add the chicken breast cubes to the sauce pan and coat the chicken with the sauce. Cook for 5 minutes on medium heat.

Nutrition Facts

Servings: 4

Amount per serving

Calories 181

% Daily Value*

Total Fat 6.3g	8%
Saturated Fat 0.7g	3%
Cholesterol 64mg	21%
Sodium 238mg	10%
Total Carbohydrate 6.7g	2%
Dietary Fiber 1g	4%
Total Sugars 0.1g	
Protein 21.8g	
Vitamin D 0mcg	0%
Calcium 31mg	2%
Iron 1mg	7%
Potassium 399mg	8%

*The % Daily Value (DV) tells you how much a nutrient in a food serving contributes to a daily diet. 2,000 calorie a day is used for general nutrition advice.

Apple Chicken Salad

Ingredients

- 1 whole roasted chicken (skin off)

- 2 green apples chopped

- 1 red onion minced

- 1/2 cup light mayonnaise

- 3 tablespoon mustard

- 1 tablespoon black pepper

Instructions

1. Wash the green apples, and chop small and set in large mixing bowl.

2. Add the minced red onion to large mixing bowl.

3. Pull the meat from the whole roasted chicken (skin off).

4. Chop the chicken small and add to large mixing bowl.

5. Add the mustard, pepper, and mayonnaise to large mixing bowl.

6. Stir all the ingredients, until well blended.

7. Serve with white/rye bread or crackers.

Nutrition Facts

Servings: 6

Amount per serving

Calories	198

	% Daily Value*
Total Fat 10.1g	13%
Saturated Fat 1.6g	8%
Cholesterol 27mg	9%
Sodium 162mg	7%
Total Carbohydrate 19.3g	7%
Dietary Fiber 3.3g	12%
Total Sugars 10.2g	
Protein 9.1g	
Vitamin D 0mcg	0%
Calcium 45mg	3%
Iron 2mg	9%
Potassium 219mg	5%

*The % Daily Value (DV) tells you how much a nutrient in a food serving contributes to a daily diet. 2,000 calorie a day is used for general nutrition advice.

Smoked Turkey Meatballs

Ingredients

- 1 pound of lean ground turkey

- 1 onion minced

- 1 tablespoon garlic powder

- 1 teaspoon black pepper

- 1/3 cup Italian bread crumbs

- 2 teaspoon fresh parsley, chopped

- 1 teaspoon Mrs. Dash®

- 1 teaspoon salt

- 2 teaspoon liquid smoke (in the seasoning aisle, used to add a smokey flavor to foods)

- 1 whole egg

- 2 teaspoon extra virgin olive oil

Instructions

1. In a large mixing bowl add the ground turkey, egg, extra virgin oil, pepper, parsley, salt, Mrs. Dash, garlic powder, minced onion, liquid smoke, and bread crumbs.

2. Stir all the ingredients together well, so that they are evenly distributed (this may take around 5 minutes).

3. In large frying pan, add 1-1/2 cups of water on medium temperature heat.

4. Roll the meatballs using your hands into small balls (golf ball size).

5. Place meatballs into the sauté pan so that they are not touching and cover with a lid and cook for around 10 minutes on each side until the meatballs are cooked thoroughly.

*Note: the water will evaporate on its own, do not drain. The water will help keep the meatballs from sticking while staying moist.

Nutrition Facts

Servings: 6

Amount per serving

Calories	**167**

	% Daily Value*
Total Fat 8.1g	**10%**
Saturated Fat 2.3g	**11%**
Cholesterol 81mg	**27%**
Sodium 557mg	**24%**
Total Carbohydrate 6.9g	**3%**
Dietary Fiber 0.7g	**3%**
Total Sugars 1.3g	
Protein 17g	
Vitamin D 3mcg	13%
Calcium 35mg	3%
Iron 2mg	10%
Potassium 305mg	6%

*The % Daily Value (DV) tells you how much a nutrient in a food serving contributes to a daily diet. 2,000 calorie a day is used for general nutrition advice.

Oven Baked Tilapia Fillets

Ingredients

- 4 (3 ounce tilapia fillets)

- 1 tablespoon unsalted butter, melted

- 2 garlic cloves minced

- 1/2 onion thinly sliced

- 1 tablespoon fresh dill

- 2 teaspoon fresh parsley, chopped

- 2 teaspoon lemon juice

- 1 teaspoon black pepper

- 2 teaspoon white cooking wine

Instructions

1. Preheat oven to 400 degrees.

2. Wash tilapia fillets under cold running water.

3. On a baking sheet place non-stick foil, add sliced onions. Place tilapia fillets on top of the sliced onions.

4. In a small bowl combine the melted butter, parsley, pepper, dill, lemon juice, and cooking wine.

5. Brush each tilapia fillet lightly with mixture.

6. Bake the tilapia fillets for 25 minutes in the preheated oven.

Nutrition Facts

Servings: 4

Amount per serving

Calories 117

% Daily Value*

Total Fat 3.7g	5%
Saturated Fat 2.2g	11%
Cholesterol 49mg	16%
Sodium 149mg	6%
Total Carbohydrate 4.2g	2%
Dietary Fiber 0.6g	2%
Total Sugars 0.7g	
Protein 16.4g	
Vitamin D 2mcg	10%
Calcium 39mg	3%
Iron 1mg	8%
Potassium 66mg	1%

*The % Daily Value (DV) tells you how much a nutrient in a food serving contributes to a daily diet. 2,000 calorie a day is used for general nutrition advice.

Erica Amber Hatcher, RD, LDN

Black Bean Turkey Sliders

Ingredients

- 1 pound ground turkey

- 1 cup frozen sweet corn

- 1/4 cup canned black beans (drained and rinsed)

- 1/2 onion minced

- 2 garlic cloves minced

- 2 teaspoon fresh cilantro chopped

- 1/4 teaspoon salt

- 1 teaspoon black pepper

- 1 teaspoon cayenne pepper

- 2 tablespoon extra virgin olive oil

- Non-stick cooking spray

- Pack of 8 mini hamburger buns

Instructions

1. Add ground turkey, corn, black beans, onion, garlic, salt, pepper, olive oil, cilantro to a large mixing bowl.

2. Blend until all ingredients are mixed thoroughly.

3. In frying pan oil pan with non-stick cooking spray on medium temperature .

4. Place small size sliders (3 ounces each) in pan. Cook for 8 minutes on both sides.

5. Place sliders on toasted mini hamburger buns.

Nutrition Facts

Servings: 8

Amount per serving

Calories 302

% Daily Value*

Total Fat 12.7g	**16%**
Saturated Fat 1.6g	**8%**
Cholesterol 58mg	**19%**
Sodium 460mg	**20%**
Total Carbohydrate 29g	**11%**
Dietary Fiber 2.6g	**9%**
Total Sugars 3.8g	
Protein 20.8g	
Vitamin D 0mcg	0%
Calcium 63mg	5%
Iron 3mg	18%
Potassium 304mg	6%

*The % Daily Value (DV) tells you how much a nutrient in a food serving contributes to a daily diet. 2,000 calorie a day is used for general nutrition advice.

Spaghetti

Ingredients

- 1 pound thin spaghetti noodles

- 1/2 cup green onions chopped

- 1 pound extra lean ground beef (90/20)

- 1 cup cherry tomatoes, sliced in half

- 2 garlic cloves minced

- 3 teaspoon fresh basil chopped

- 1/2 green pepper chopped

- 1/4 tsp salt

- 1 teaspoon black pepper

- 2 teaspoon extra virgin olive oil

- 2 teaspoon oregano

- 1/4 cup Parmesan cheese grated

Instructions

1. Boil water and add pasta. Boil for 9 minutes or al dente. Add 1 tsp. extra virgin oil to water to prevent pasta from sticking.

2. Drain noodles well in a colander under running cold water to prevent further cooking.

3. In a large sauce pan add ground beef until fully cooked and drain out excess oil.

4. Return ground beef to a low heat.

5. Add garlic, green onions, basil, salt, pepper, oregano, green peppers, tomatoes, and sauté on medium heat for 5 minutes.

6. Remove from stove and add to serving bowl and combine with noodles. Add remainder of 1 teaspoon extra virgin olive oil and Parmesan cheese.

Nutrition Facts

Servings: 6

Amount per serving

Calories	227

% Daily Value*

Total Fat 8.7g	**11%**
Saturated Fat 3.8g	**19%**
Cholesterol 64mg	**21%**
Sodium 236mg	**10%**
Total Carbohydrate 3.5g	**1%**
Dietary Fiber 1.1g	**4%**
Total Sugars 1.3g	
Protein 23.6g	
Vitamin D 0mcg	0%
Calcium 111mg	9%
Iron 7mg	36%
Potassium 393mg	8%

*The % Daily Value (DV) tells you how much a nutrient in a food serving contributes to a daily diet. 2,000 calorie a day is used for general nutrition advice.

Erica Amber Hatcher, RD, LDN

Turkey Kielbasa

Ingredients

- 1 pound turkey kielbasa

- 1 green pepper (chopped)

- 1 red pepper (chopped)

- 1 yellow pepper (chopped)

- 2 garlic cloves minced

- 1 yellow onion (diced)

- 1 teaspoon Mrs. Dash®

- 1 teaspoon black pepper

- 2 teaspoon extra virgin olive oil

Instructions

1. Slice turkey kielbasa (thinly sliced).

2. In a large sauté pan add 2 teaspoon extra virgin olive oil.

3. Allow pan to get hot (approximately 2-3 minutes).

4. Add onions, green pepper, yellow pepper, red pepper, and garlic.

5. Saute on medium heat for approximately 8 minutes or until tender and onion is transparent.

6. Add Mrs. Dash® and pepper to season.

7. Add turkey kielbasa and cook on low heat for approximately 15 minutes. Stir constantly.

8. Remove kielbasa from heat and place on large plate for serving.

Nutrition Facts

Servings: 4

Amount per serving

Calories 182

% Daily Value*

Total Fat 8.7g	11%
Saturated Fat 3.4g	17%
Cholesterol 28mg	9%
Sodium 571mg	25%
Total Carbohydrate 12g	4%
Dietary Fiber 2.1g	7%
Total Sugars 5.4g	
Protein 19.7g	
Vitamin D 0mcg	0%
Calcium 22mg	2%
Iron 2mg	12%
Potassium 262mg	6%

*The % Daily Value (DV) tells you how much a nutrient in a food serving contributes to a daily diet. 2,000 calorie a day is used for general nutrition advice.

Shrimp Scampi

Ingredients

- 2 tablespoons unsalted butter, softened

- 1/4 cup extra virgin olive oil

- 1 tablespoon minced garlic

- 1 tablespoon minced shallots

- 2 tablespoons minced fresh chives

- 1/4 teaspoon salt

- 1 teaspoon freshly ground black pepper

- 1/2 teaspoon paprika

- 1 pound large shrimp, peeled and deveined

Instructions

1. Preheat grill for high heat.

2. In a large bowl, mix together softened butter, olive oil, garlic, shallots, chives, salt, pepper, and paprika. Add the shrimp, and toss to coat.

3. Lightly oil grill grate. Cook the shrimp as close to the flame as possible for 2 to 3 minutes per side, or until opaque.

Nutrition Facts

Servings: 6

Amount per serving

Calories	172

	% Daily Value*
Total Fat 12.3g	16%
Saturated Fat 3.6g	18%
Cholesterol 118mg	39%
Sodium 219mg	10%
Total Carbohydrate 2.5g	1%
Dietary Fiber 0.2g	1%
Total Sugars 0.1g	
Protein 14.5g	
Vitamin D 3mcg	13%
Calcium 7mg	1%
Iron 0mg	1%
Potassium 24mg	1%

*The % Daily Value (DV) tells you how much a nutrient in a food serving contributes to a daily diet. 2,000 calorie a day is used for general nutrition advice.

Grilled Chicken Fiesta Salad

Ingredients

- 2 boneless skinless chicken breasts (sliced)

- 1 tsp extra virgin olive oil

- 1/2 cup diced green and red peppers

- 2 teaspoon diced red onion

- 1/4 teaspoon salt

- 1 teaspoon chili powder

- 1/2 teaspoon ground cumin

- 1/2 teaspoon oregano

- 1/2 cup frozen yellow corn kernels, thawed

- 2 cups fresh romaine lettuce (washed and cut)

- 1/4 cup fresh cilantro

- 1/2 avocado sliced thin

- 1 cup crispy tortilla chips (broken into pieces)

- 3 tablespoons balsamic vinaigrette

Nutrition Facts

Servings: 4

Amount per serving

Calories	**286**

	% Daily Value*
Total Fat 16.6g	21%
Saturated Fat 3.5g	18%
Cholesterol 65mg	22%
Sodium 375mg	16%
Total Carbohydrate 11.9g	4%
Dietary Fiber 3.2g	12%
Total Sugars 2.5g	
Protein 22.9g	
Vitamin D 0mcg	0%
Calcium 30mg	2%
Iron 2mg	13%
Potassium 429mg	9%

*The % Daily Value (DV) tells you how much a nutrient in a food serving contributes to a daily diet. 2,000 calorie a day is used for general nutrition advice.

Instructions

1. Clean chicken and remove any visible fat from chicken breasts. Sprinkle chicken with spices and toss and coat evenly.

2. Heat the olive oil in a large skillet; add chicken and sauté until golden brown, about 7-8 minutes. Then add the corn and sauté' for an additional 2 minutes. Remove from pan and allow to cool.

3. In a large salad bowl add the romaine lettuce, green and red peppers, red onion, cilantro and balsamic vinaigrette. Toss together.

4. Place the sauteed chicken, corn and avocado on top. Add the tortilla chips on the side edges (to prevent them from getting soft or soggy).

Asian Grilled Pork Tenderloin

Ingredients

- 6 ounces boneless pork tenderloin

- 1 tablespoon low-sodium soy sauce

- 2 teaspoons toasted sesame oil

- 1/2 teaspoon garlic clove (minced)

- 1/2 teaspoon ground ginger

- 1/4 teaspoon salt

- 1 teaspoon freshly ground black pepper

- 1/2 teaspoon chili powder

- 1 teaspoon fresh parsley chopped

Instructions

1. Preheat grill to medium heat.

2. Slice pork tenderloin diagonally into 6-8 slices.

3. In a large bowl, stir together soy sauce, sesame oil, garlic, ginger, chili powder, black pepper, and salt. Coat the pieces of pork tenderloin with the sauce mixture. Make sure the sauce is on both sides of the pork.

4. Add pieces to hot grill. Cook 3-4 minutes on each side. Make sure to cook the pork thoroughly, until it is no longer pink in the middle.

5. Sprinkle with fresh parsley. Serve immediately.

Nutrition Facts

Servings: 6

Amount per serving

Calories 57

% Daily Value*

Total Fat 2.6g	3%
Saturated Fat 0.6g	3%
Cholesterol 21mg	7%
Sodium 262mg	11%
Total Carbohydrate 0.7g	0%
Dietary Fiber 0.2g	1%
Total Sugars 0.2g	
Protein 7.7g	
Vitamin D 0mcg	0%
Calcium 5mg	0%
Iron 0mg	3%
Potassium 132mg	3%

*The % Daily Value (DV) tells you how much a nutrient in a food serving contributes to a daily diet. 2,000 calorie a day is used for general nutrition advice.

Erica Amber Hatcher, RD, LDN

Crab Fried Rice

Ingredients

- 6 cups cooked rice

- 2 eggs

- 1 1/2 tablespoons fish sauce

- 3 cloves chopped garlic

- 2-3 chopped green onion

- 1/3 cup shredded carrots

- 2 tablespoons diced yellow onion

- 3-5 tablespoons cooking oil

- 1 teaspoon ground black pepper

- 1 teaspoon chopped cilantro

- 1 cup lump crab meat

Instructions

1. Over medium to high heat, add 3 tablespoons of oil to a wok or a large pot. You'll need room to stir the rice around. Add chopped garlic to the oil, and the yellow onion. When the garlic begins to brown, add the rice and shredded carrots. Stir and mix the rice with the oil. Add crab meat and stir again.

2. Make room in the middle of the wok. Add a teaspoon of oil and crack the egg into the spot. Scramble the egg to cook it. Then incorporate the egg into the rest of the fried rice. Repeat the same steps to add another egg.

3. Add fish sauce and ground black pepper and turn off the heat. Add the chopped green onions. Add in the cilantro leaves and lump crab meat, stir gently and serve.

4. Tip: Drier rice gives you fluffy fried rice as opposed to gummy/mushy fried rice. Cook rice with about 10% less water than normal to get firmer rice.

Nutrition Facts

Servings: 6

Amount per serving

Calories 770

% Daily Value*

Total Fat 9.9g	13%
Saturated Fat 1.8g	9%
Cholesterol 57mg	19%
Sodium 412mg	18%
Total Carbohydrate 150.3g	55%
Dietary Fiber 2.9g	10%
Total Sugars 1.1g	
Protein 16.3g	
Vitamin D 5mcg	26%
Calcium 89mg	7%
Iron 9mg	48%
Potassium 294mg	6%

*The % Daily Value (DV) tells you how much a nutrient in a food serving contributes to a daily diet. 2,000 calorie a day is used for general nutrition advice.

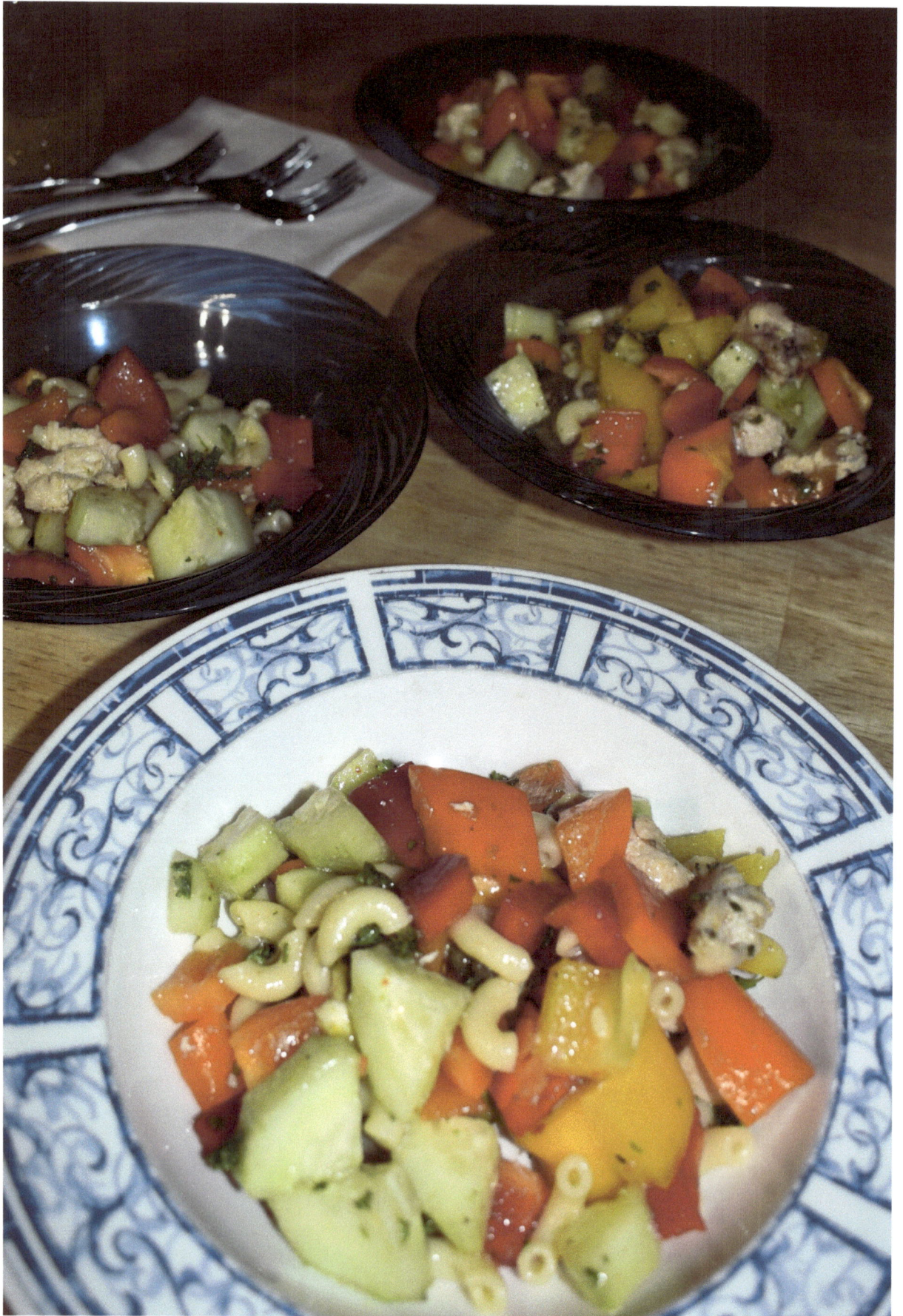

Roasted Chicken Pasta

Ingredients

- 1 cup roasted chicken skin off

- 8 ounce elbow macaroni

- 1 red bell pepper

- 1 yellow bell pepper

- 1 orange bell pepper

- 1 teaspoon capers

- 1/2 cucumber diced

- 1/3 cup Italian salad dressing

- 1 teaspoon cayenne pepper

- 1 tablespoon fresh parsley

Instructions

1. Pull chicken from bones; chop into small pieces (make sure to remove all the skin). Boil a large pot of water, add pasta for 9 minutes or soft, drain under cold water.

2. Dice yellow, red, orange pepper, cucumber and red onion.

3. Add above ingredients to a large mixing bowl. Add in Italian dressing, cayenne pepper, capers, and parley.

4. Chill at least 6-8 hours serve.

Nutrition Facts

Servings: 4

Amount per serving

Calories	380

	% Daily Value*
Total Fat 9.5g	12%
Saturated Fat 1.9g	9%
Cholesterol 46mg	15%
Sodium 66mg	3%
Total Carbohydrate 54.4g	20%
Dietary Fiber 3.6g	13%
Total Sugars 7.2g	
Protein 19.7g	
Vitamin D 0mcg	0%
Calcium 41mg	3%
Iron 3mg	17%
Potassium 504mg	11%

*The % Daily Value (DV) tells you how much a nutrient in a food serving contributes to a daily diet. 2,000 calorie a day is used for general nutrition advice.

Fettuccine Alfredo

Ingredients

- 12 ounces fettuccine, uncooked

- 3 tablespoons unsalted butter

- 2 garlic cloves

- 1/4 cup orange bell pepper

- 1/4 cup green bell pepper

- 2 tablespoons all-purpose white flour

- 1/4 cup white wine

- 3/4 cup low-sodium vegetable broth

- 3/4 cup non-dairy creamer

- 2 teaspoons dried basil

- 1/4 cup grated parmesan cheese

- 1 teaspoon red pepper flakes

- 1 teaspoon onion powder

Nutrition Facts

Servings: 6

Amount per serving

Calories 248

	% Daily Value*
Total Fat 7.5g	10%
Saturated Fat 4g	20%
Cholesterol 58mg	19%
Sodium 68mg	3%
Total Carbohydrate 36.2g	13%
Dietary Fiber 0.6g	2%
Total Sugars 1.5g	
Protein 7.6g	
Vitamin D 4mcg	20%
Calcium 29mg	2%
Iron 2mg	13%
Potassium 178mg	4%

*The % Daily Value (DV) tells you how much a nutrient in a food serving contributes to a daily diet. 2,000 calorie a day is used for general nutrition advice.

Instructions

1. Mince garlic and slice red bell pepper, and green bell pepper. Cook fettuccine in boiling water for 10 minutes (usually al dente). Drain and set aside.

2. Melt butter in a medium saucepan. Add garlic and red, and green bell pepper. Sauté 1 to 2 minutes until vegetables are soft.

3. Slowly stir flour into the pan. Cook 1 minute until smooth. Add wine gradually, stirring until smooth.

4. Add broth, nondairy creamer, basil, onion powder, red pepper flakes, and black pepper. Stir to blend.

5. Gradually add Parmesan cheese. Reduce heat to low and cook 5 to 7 minutes until mixture starts to simmer. Toss the sauce with the drained fettuccine.

Oven Fried Chicken with

Honey Mustard Glaze

Ingredients

- 8 boneless, skinless chicken thighs

- 2 teaspoon Mrs. Dash® seasoning

- 2 teaspoon smoked paprika

- 2 teaspoon garlic powder

- 2 teaspoon onion powder

- 1 teaspoon black pepper

- 1 teaspoon red pepper flakes

- 2 large eggs

- 1/4 cup non dairy creamer

- 1-1/2 cups flour

- Non-stick cooking spray

- 2 tablespoons fresh chopped parsley flakes

For the honey mustard glaze

- 1/4 cup light mayo

- 2 tablespoons honey

- 1 tablespoon yellow mustard

- 1 tablespoon Dijon mustard

Nutrition Facts

Servings: 8

Amount per serving

Calories	456
	% Daily Value*
Total Fat 17.9g	**23%**
Saturated Fat 4.2g	**21%**
Cholesterol 179mg	**60%**
Sodium 225mg	**10%**
Total Carbohydrate 24.8g	**9%**
Dietary Fiber 1.2g	**4%**
Total Sugars 5g	
Protein 22g	
Vitamin D 4mcg	22%
Calcium 40mg	3%
Iron 3mg	19%
Potassium 447mg	10%

*The % Daily Value (DV) tells you how much a nutrient in a food serving contributes to a daily diet. 2,000 calorie a day is used for general nutrition advice.

Instructions

1. Preheat oven to 375 degrees. To make the honey mustard glaze, whisk mayo, honey and mustard in a small bowl and set aside.

2. Wash the chicken thighs, take off all the skin on the chicken.

3. Season chicken thighs with onion powder, Mrs. Dash®, garlic powder, red pepper flakes, smoked paprika, and black pepper.

4. In a large bowl whisk together eggs, non-dairy creamer.

5. Working one at a time, dredge the chicken in the flour, then into the egg mixture pressing to coat.

6. Place chicken onto a baking sheet covered in non stick foil. Spray non-stick cooking spray on each piece of chicken.

7. Bake 35-40 minutes until the crust is golden brown and the chicken is cooked through.

8. Serve immediately with the honey mustard glaze. Garnish with parsley if desired.

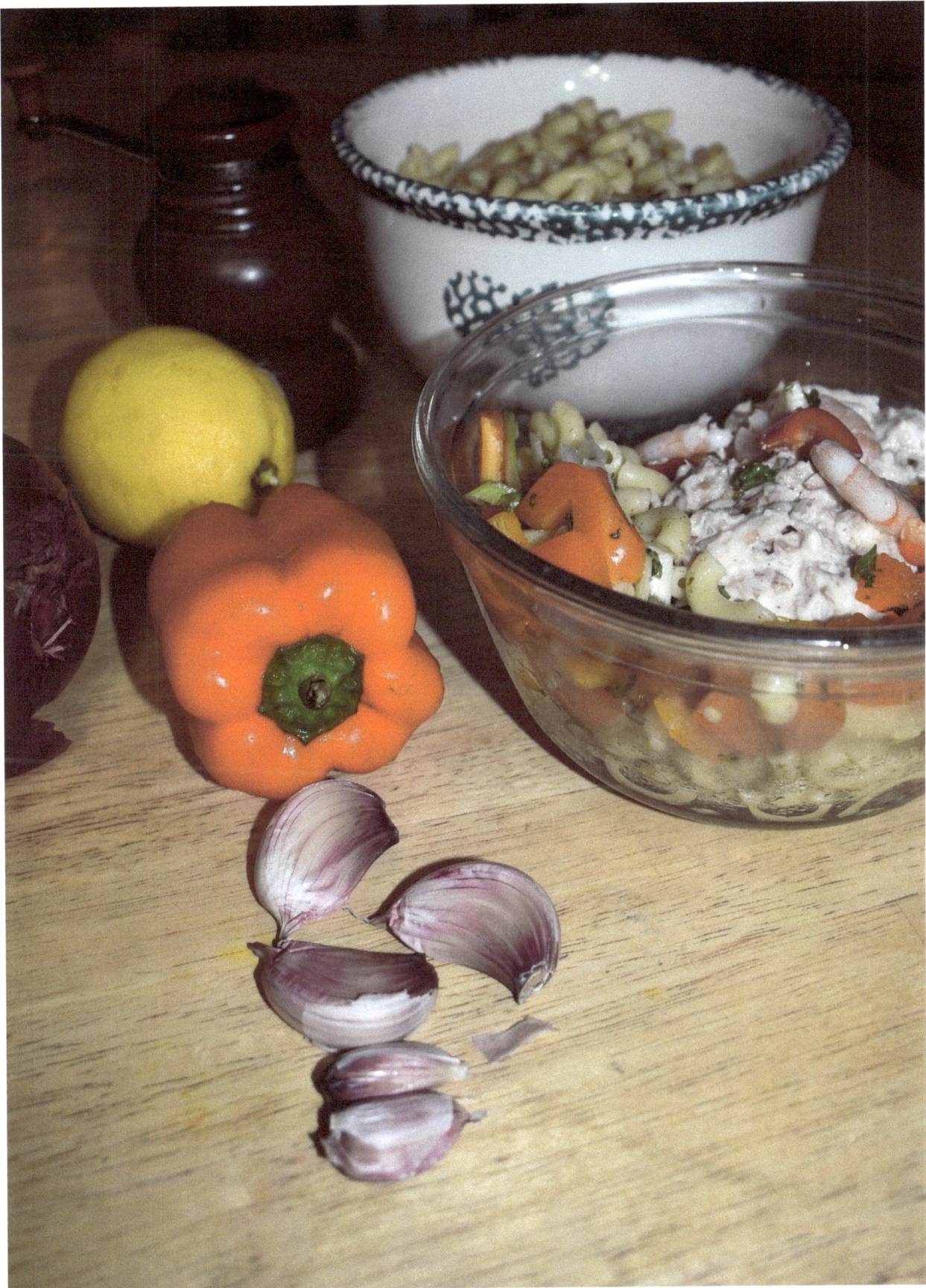

Yacht Club Seafood Salad

Ingredients

- 1/4 cup diced onion

- 1/4 cup red pepper diced

- 1/4 cup yellow pepper diced

- 1/4 cup orange pepper diced

- 4 ounces fresh crab meat (Lump)

- 1 can albacore tuna packed in water

- 1/2 lb shrimp steamed and diced

- 1/2 cup light mayo

- 1 tablespoon mustard

- 1 tablespoon fresh parsley

- 1/4 tablespoon Old Bay® seasoning

- 1 tablespoon black pepper

- 1 tsp. paprika

- 12 oz elbow macaroni boiled 9 minutes or until tender

Nutrition Facts

Servings: 6

Amount per serving

Calories — **354**

	% Daily Value*
Total Fat 7.3g	9%
Saturated Fat 1.2g	6%
Cholesterol 100mg	33%
Sodium 458mg	20%
Total Carbohydrate 49.1g	18%
Dietary Fiber 3g	11%
Total Sugars 2.2g	
Protein 21.6g	
Vitamin D 0mcg	0%
Calcium 134mg	10%
Iron 3mg	17%
Potassium 343mg	7%

*The % Daily Value (DV) tells you how much a nutrient in a food serving contributes to a daily diet. 2,000 calorie a day is used for general nutrition advice.

Instructions

1. Dice onion, red, yellow and orange pepper. Place in large container. Boil water for shrimp, gently cook shrimp in boiling water for about 3 minutes. Make sure you remove all shells. Cool shrimp and cut into pieces. Drain tuna and dice add to peppers and onion. Once shrimp is cooled, add to mixture. Add lump crab meat, mayo, black pepper, mustard, Old Bay®, and paprika. Mix all ingredients gently. Add elbow macaroni after it has cooled. Garnish with parsley and chill.

2. Serve seafood salad cold.

Warning: AVOID if you have an allergy to shell fish!!!!!

Low Sodium Chipped Beef Dip

Ingredients

- 8 ounces light cream cheese

- 8 ounces light chive and onion cream cheese (tub)

- 10 ounces low sodium chipped beef, chopped fine

- 1 tablespoon Worcestershire sauce

- 1 teaspoon garlic powder

Instructions

1. Mix all ingredients well. Chill and serve with cracker

Nutrition Facts

Servings: 6

Amount per serving

Calories 268

% Daily Value*

Total Fat 26.4g	34%
Saturated Fat 16.6g	83%
Cholesterol 83mg	28%
Sodium 252mg	11%
Total Carbohydrate 2.9g	1%
Dietary Fiber 0.1g	0%
Total Sugars 0.8g	
Protein 5.8g	
Vitamin D 0mcg	0%
Calcium 61mg	5%
Iron 1mg	5%
Potassium 95mg	2%

*The % Daily Value (DV) tells you how much a nutrient in a food serving contributes to a daily diet. 2,000 calorie a day is used for general nutrition advice.

Sauteed Beef Tips

Ingredients

- 1 small onion

- 1/2 medium tomato

- 1/2 medium green bell pepper

- 1/2 medium red bell pepper

- 8 ounces lean stewing beef

- 2 tablespoons extra virgin oil

- 1/4 teaspoon salt

- 1/8 teaspoon black pepper

- 1 small jalapeno chopped

Instructions

1. Thinly slice onion. Chop tomato, green and red bell peppers. Cut beef into small cubes.

2. Sauté onion and oil in a skillet until the onion is slightly brown. Add beef and tomatoes.

3. When partially cooked, add bell peppers, salt and pepper.

4. Continue cooking until meat is tender.

Nutrition Facts

Servings: 3

Amount per serving

Calories 244

	% Daily Value*
Total Fat 13.9g	18%
Saturated Fat 1.3g	7%
Cholesterol 0mg	0%
Sodium 286mg	12%
Total Carbohydrate 5.9g	2%
Dietary Fiber 1.4g	5%
Total Sugars 3.2g	
Protein 24.7g	
Vitamin D 0mcg	0%
Calcium 13mg	1%
Iron 1mg	3%
Potassium 121mg	3%

*The % Daily Value (DV) tells you how much a nutrient in a food serving contributes to a daily diet. 2,000 calorie a day is used for general nutrition advice.

Oven Roasted Brussels Sprouts

Ingredients

- 1 pound brussels sprouts, rinsed, ends trimmed

- 1 tablespoon minced garlic (about 3 cloves)

- 1 teaspoon lemon juice

- 2 tablespoons olive oil

- 1/4 tsp. salt

- 1 teaspoon freshly ground black pepper

- 1/4 cup freshly grated parmesan cheese (optional)

Instructions

1. Preheat oven to 350°F.

2. Toss sprouts with garlic, lemon juice, olive oil, salt. Spread onto a roasting pan: Place Brussels sprouts in a large bowl. Toss with garlic and lemon juice. Toss with olive oil so that the sprouts are well coated.

3. Spread the Brussels sprouts out on a flat roasting pan covered with non stick foil in a single layer with plenty of space between the sprouts. Sprinkle with salt, and black pepper.

4. Roast in oven: Put Brussels sprouts in oven on top rack, roast for 30 minutes, stirring the sprouts about halfway through the cooking.

5. The sprouts should be nicely browned, with some of the outside leaves crunchy, the interior should be cooked through.

6. Sprinkle with Parmesan cheese.

Nutrition Facts

Servings: 4

Amount per serving

Calories 159

% Daily Value*

Total Fat 10.4g	13%
Saturated Fat 3.2g	16%
Cholesterol 10mg	3%
Sodium 306mg	13%
Total Carbohydrate 11.9g	4%
Dietary Fiber 4.4g	16%
Total Sugars 2.5g	
Protein 8.6g	
Vitamin D 0mcg	0%
Calcium 170mg	13%
Iron 2mg	9%
Potassium 457mg	10%

*The % Daily Value (DV) tells you how much a nutrient in a food serving contributes to a daily diet. 2,000 calorie a day is used for general nutrition advice.

Roasted Vegetables

Ingredients

- 2 tablespoons olive oil, divided

- 1 large yam, peeled and cut into 1 inch pieces

- 1 large parsnip, peeled and cut into 1 inch pieces

- 1 cup baby carrots

- 1 small onion diced

- 1 zucchini, cut into 1 inch slices

- 1 bunch fresh asparagus, trimmed and cut into 1 inch pieces

- 1 red pepper diced

- 2 cloves garlic, minced

- 1/2 cup chopped fresh basil

- 1/2 teaspoon kosher salt

- 1/2 teaspoon ground black pepper

Instructions

1. Preheat oven to 425 degrees. Grease 2 baking sheets with 1 tablespoon olive oil.

Nutrition Facts	
Servings: 4	
Amount per serving	
Calories	**135**
	% Daily Value*
Total Fat 7.4g	9%
Saturated Fat 1g	5%
Cholesterol 0mg	0%
Sodium 305mg	13%
Total Carbohydrate 17.4g	6%
Dietary Fiber 4g	14%
Total Sugars 5.1g	
Protein 2.1g	
Vitamin D 0mcg	0%
Calcium 40mg	3%
Iron 1mg	6%
Potassium 486mg	10%

*The % Daily Value (DV) tells you how much a nutrient in a food serving contributes to a daily diet. 2,000 calorie a day is used for general nutrition advice.

2. Place the yams, parsnips, onion, red pepper and carrots onto the baking sheets. Bake in the preheated oven for 30 minutes, then add the zucchini and asparagus, and drizzle with the remaining 1 tablespoon of olive oil. Continue baking until all of the vegetables are tender, about 30 minutes more. Once tender, remove from the oven, and allow to cool for 30 minutes on the baking sheet.

3. Toss the garlic, basil, salt, and pepper in a large bowl until combined. Add the roasted vegetables, and toss to mix. Serve at room temperature or cold.

Vegetable Linguine Salad

Ingredients

- 1 pound linguine noodles

- 1/2 cup fresh broccoli spears (chopped)

- 1 zucchini (chopped small)

- 1 cup diced green onions

- 2 garlic cloves minced

- 3 teaspoon fresh cilantro chopped

- 1/4 teaspoon salt

- 1 teaspoon black pepper

- 1 summer squash, chopped small

- 1 cup lite Italian dressing

- 1/4 cup parmesan cheese grated

- 2 tsp extra virgin olive oil

Instructions

1. Boil water and add pasta, boil for 9 minutes or al dente. Add olive oil to water to prevent pasta from sticking.

2. Drain noodles well in a colander under running cold water to prevent further cooking. Let noodles drain for 10 minutes.

3. In a large mixing bowl combine the drained noodles and the rest of the ingredients, except for the parmesan cheese, stir ingredients well.

4. Add Parmesan cheese and refrigerate for at least 1 hour.

Nutrition Facts

Servings: 8

Amount per serving

Calories 340

% Daily Value*

Total Fat 10.2g	**13%**
Saturated Fat 2.6g	**13%**
Cholesterol 10mg	**3%**
Sodium 464mg	**20%**
Total Carbohydrate 47.8g	**17%**
Dietary Fiber 3.5g	**12%**
Total Sugars 4.5g	
Protein 12.8g	
Vitamin D 0mcg	0%
Calcium 152mg	12%
Iron 2mg	13%
Potassium 140mg	3%

*The % Daily Value (DV) tells you how much a nutrient in a food serving contributes to a daily diet. 2,000 calorie a day is used for general nutrition advice.

E's Family Favorite Fried Potatoes and Onion

Ingredients

- About 1/2 cup of extra virgin olive oil

- 2 pounds of russet potatoes (about 4 to 5), peeled and diced (Make sure you have soaked the potatoes at least 4 hours prior to cooking, to release the potassium from the potatoes)

- 1-1/2 cup of finely chopped sweet onion

- 2 garlic cloves minced

- 1 teaspoon garlic powder

- 1 tablespoon dried parsley flakes

- 1/4 teaspoon salt

Instructions

1. In a large pot heat oil, to test temperature of the oil add 1 diced potato. Once oil is ready add potatoes, stir to ensure potatoes are coated with the oil, cover with lid and allow to cook for 8 minutes. Next add onion, minced garlic and garlic powder, salt and dried parsley flakes. Stir frequently then turn down the heat slightly, let cook for around 15 – 20 minutes. Keep turning the potatoes so they can cook evenly, around 5 minute intervals.

2. Serve garnish with more parsley flakes if desired.

Nutrition Facts	
Servings: 6	
Amount per serving	
Calories	**273**
	% Daily Value*
Total Fat 18.9g	**24%**
Saturated Fat 2.7g	**14%**
Cholesterol 0mg	**0%**
Sodium 107mg	**5%**
Total Carbohydrate 25.7g	**9%**
Dietary Fiber 4.1g	**15%**
Total Sugars 3g	
Protein 2.9g	
Vitamin D 0mcg	0%
Calcium 22mg	2%
Iron 1mg	5%
Potassium 631mg	13%

*The % Daily Value (DV) tells you how much a nutrient in a food serving contributes to a daily diet. 2,000 calorie a day is used for general nutrition advice.

Beverages

Energy Smoothie

Ingredients

- 1 banana

- 1 cup frozen strawberries

- 1 cup frozen blueberries

- 1 cup frozen cherries

- 4 ice cubes

- 1/2 cup cranberry juice juice

- 1/4 cup pineapple juice

- 3/4 cup vanilla Greek yogurt

- 1/2 teaspoon honey

Instructions

1. Place the banana, strawberries, blueberries, cherries, and ice cubes into a blender. Pour in the orange juice, vanilla yogurt, and honey. Puree until smooth.

Nutrition Facts

Servings: 4

Amount per serving

Calories 132

% Daily Value*

Total Fat 1.2g	2%
Saturated Fat 0.6g	3%
Cholesterol 2mg	1%
Sodium 16mg	1%
Total Carbohydrate 27g	10%
Dietary Fiber 3.6g	13%
Total Sugars 18.8g	
Protein 4.8g	
Vitamin D 0mcg	0%
Calcium 58mg	4%
Iron 1mg	6%
Potassium 299mg	6%

*The % Daily Value (DV) tells you how much a nutrient in a food serving contributes to a daily diet. 2,000 calorie a day is used for general nutrition advice.

Sunset Juice

Ingredients

- 1 large apple, quartered
- 1 cup pineapple chunks (canned)
- 3 large carrots, ends trimmed
- 2 teaspoons fresh ginger
- 2 large stalks celery
- 1/2 medium beet
- 2 tbsp fresh chopped mint

Instructions

1. Juice the apple, pineapple, carrots, ginger, celery, mint and beet in a juice machine.

Nutrition Facts

Servings: 4

Amount per serving

Calories	85

	% Daily Value*
Total Fat 0.3g	0%
Saturated Fat 0g	0%
Cholesterol 0mg	0%
Sodium 65mg	3%
Total Carbohydrate 21.1g	8%
Dietary Fiber 4.1g	15%
Total Sugars 13.8g	
Protein 1.3g	
Vitamin D 0mcg	0%
Calcium 40mg	3%
Iron 1mg	6%
Potassium 393mg	8%

*The % Daily Value (DV) tells you how much a nutrient in a food serving contributes to a daily diet. 2,000 calorie a day is used for general nutrition advice.

Desserts

Rice Pudding

Ingredients

- 1 cup long-grain rice

- 2 cups water

- 2 cups rice milk (rice dream)

- 1/2 cup sugar substitute (Splenda®)

- 1/2 cup cinnamon

- 1/2 cup nutmeg

- 2 eggs, beaten

- 2 teaspoons vanilla extract

Instructions

1. Bring 2 cups water to a boil in medium saucepan.

2. Add rice; return to a boil.

3. Reduce heat to low, cover and cook 20 minutes until liquid is absorbed.

4. Stir in rice milk, sugar substitute, cinnamon and nutmeg.

5. Cook over medium heat, stirring frequently, for about 15 minutes until most of the liquid is absorbed.

6. Meanwhile, beat together eggs and vanilla together in a bowl. Add slowly to 2 cups of rice pudding to egg mixture, and then stir egg mixture into remaining pudding.

7. Cook, stirring constantly, for 2 to 3 minutes until thickened.

Nutrition Facts

Servings: 4

Amount per serving

Calories	**490**

	% Daily Value*
Total Fat 8.5g	11%
Saturated Fat 4.3g	22%
Cholesterol 82mg	27%
Sodium 83mg	4%
Total Carbohydrate 91.5g	33%
Dietary Fiber 10.7g	38%
Total Sugars 28.6g	
Protein 7.6g	
Vitamin D 8mcg	39%
Calcium 201mg	15%
Iron 4mg	22%
Potassium 227mg	5%

*The % Daily Value (DV) tells you how much a nutrient in a food serving contributes to a daily diet. 2,000 calorie a day is used for general nutrition advice.

Easy Pretzel Salad

Ingredients

- 2 cups crushed pretzels

- 3/4 cup unsalted butter, melted

- 2 teaspoons Splenda® or white sugar

- 1 (8 ounce) package light cream cheese

- 3/4 cup white sugar

- 4 1/2 ounces frozen whipped topping, thawed

- 1 (6 ounce) package strawberry flavored Jell-O®

- 2 cups boiling water

- 2 (10 ounce) packages frozen strawberries

Instructions

1. Preheat oven to 400 degrees F.

2. In a medium bowl, mix crushed pretzels, margarine and sugar.

3. Press crushed pretzel mixture into the bottom of a 9x13 inch baking dish, and bake in the preheated oven 8 minutes. Remove from heat and allow to cool.

4. Blend together the cream cheese and Splenda/ sugar. Fold in whipped topping and spread evenly over cooled pretzel mixture.

5. In a medium bowl, dissolve the strawberry flavored gelatin in boiling water. Mix in strawberries and set aside to cool for 15 minutes.

6. Pour gelatin mixture over cream cheese mixture and refrigerate until set, about 6 hours, and serve.

Nutrition Facts

Servings: 6

Amount per serving

Calories	**716**

	% Daily Value*
Total Fat 41.5g	**53%**
Saturated Fat 25.9g	**130%**
Cholesterol 119mg	**40%**
Sodium 745mg	**32%**
Total Carbohydrate 82.1g	**30%**
Dietary Fiber 2.6g	**9%**
Total Sugars 59.7g	
Protein 8.9g	
Vitamin D 16mcg	79%
Calcium 78mg	6%
Iron 2mg	12%
Potassium 116mg	2%

*The % Daily Value (DV) tells you how much a nutrient in a food serving contributes to a daily diet. 2,000 calorie a day is used for general nutrition advice.

Lemon Bars

Ingredients

- 1-1/2 cups all-purpose flour

- 2/3 cup confectioners sugar

- 3/4 cup butter or margarine, softened

- 3 eggs

- 1 1/2 cups Splenda or white sugar

- 3 tablespoons all-purpose flour

- 1/4 cup lemon juice

- 1/3 cup confectioners sugar for decoration

Instructions

1. Preheat the oven to 375 degrees F. Grease a 9x13 inch baking pan.

2. Combine the flour, 2/3 cup confectioners sugar, and butter. Pat dough into prepared pan.

3. Bake for 20 minutes in the preheated oven, until slightly golden. While the crust is baking, whisk together eggs, Splenda /white sugar, flour, and lemon juice until frothy. Pour this lemon mixture over the hot crust.

4. Return to the preheated oven for an additional 20 to 25 minutes, or until light golden brown. Cool on a wire rack. Dust the top with confectioners sugar. Cut into squares.

Nutrition Facts

Servings: 6

Amount per serving

Calories 615

% Daily Value*

Total Fat 25.6g	33%
Saturated Fat 15.4g	77%
Cholesterol 143mg	48%
Sodium 197mg	9%
Total Carbohydrate 93.5g	34%
Dietary Fiber 0.9g	3%
Total Sugars 63.6g	
Protein 6.4g	
Vitamin D 24mcg	118%
Calcium 24mg	2%
Iron 2mg	11%
Potassium 83mg	2%

*The % Daily Value (DV) tells you how much a nutrient in a food serving contributes to a daily diet. 2,000 calorie a day is used for general nutrition advice.

Baked Apple Crisp

Ingredients

- 4 cups sliced apples

- 1 teaspoon ground cinnamon

- 1/2 cup water

- 1 cup white sugar

- 1/4 cup unsalted butter

- 3/4 cup all-purpose flour

Instructions

1. Preheat oven to 350 degrees. Grease an 8x8 inch baking dish.

2. Place apples in prepared dish. Sprinkle with cinnamon. Pour water over all. In a bowl, cream together sugar and butter. Blend in flour slowly. Sprinkle mixture evenly over apples.

3. Bake in preheated oven 30 to 40 minutes, until apples are tender and crust is golden.

Nutrition Facts

Servings: 4

Amount per serving

Calories 492

	% Daily Value*
Total Fat 12.2g	16%
Saturated Fat 7.3g	37%
Cholesterol 31mg	10%
Sodium 85mg	4%
Total Carbohydrate 99.2g	36%
Dietary Fiber 6.3g	23%
Total Sugars 73.3g	
Protein 3.2g	
Vitamin D 8mcg	40%
Calcium 15mg	1%
Iron 2mg	12%
Potassium 270mg	6%

*The % Daily Value (DV) tells you how much a nutrient in a food serving contributes to a daily diet. 2,000 calorie a day is used for general nutrition advice.

Miscellaneous

Chicken Stock

Ingredients

- 1 whole free-range chicken (about 3-1/2 pounds), rinsed, giblets discarded

- 2 carrots, cut in large chunks

- 3 celery stalks, cut in large chunks

- 2 large white onions, quartered

- 1 head of garlic, halved

- 1/4 teaspoon thyme

- 2 bay leaves

- 1 teaspoon black pepper

Instructions

1. Place the chicken and vegetables in a large stockpot over medium heat. Pour in only enough cold water to cover (about 3 quarts); too much will make the broth taste weak. Toss in the thyme, bay leaves, and black pepper, and allow it to slowly come to a boil. Lower the heat to medium-low and gently simmer for 1 to 1-1/2 hours, partially covered, until the chicken is done. As it cooks, skim any impurities that rise to the surface; add a little more water if necessary to keep the chicken covered while simmering.

2. Carefully remove the chicken to a cutting board. When it is cool enough to handle, discard the skin and bones; hand-shred the meat into a storage container.

3. Carefully strain the stock through a fine sieve into another pot to remove the vegetable solids. Use the stock immediately or if you plan on storing it, place the pot in a sink full of ice water and stir to cool down the stock. Cover and refrigerate for up to one week or freeze. Yield: 2 quarts.

Nutrition Facts

Servings: 6

Amount per serving

Calories 322

% Daily Value*

Total Fat 20.3g	**26%**
Saturated Fat 5.8g	**29%**
Cholesterol 100mg	**33%**
Sodium 123mg	**5%**
Total Carbohydrate 8.1g	**3%**
Dietary Fiber 2g	**7%**
Total Sugars 3.3g	
Protein 25.9g	
Vitamin D 0mcg	0%
Calcium 32mg	2%
Iron 1mg	4%
Potassium 174mg	4%

*The % Daily Value (DV) tells you how much a nutrient in a food serving contributes to a daily diet. 2,000 calorie a day is used for general nutrition advice.

Homemade BBQ Sauce

Ingredients

- 1 tablespoon extra virgin olive oil

- 2 cloves garlic, minced

- 1/2 onion, diced

- 1 cup ketchup

- 1/3 cup molasses

- 1/3 cup brown sugar

- 4 tablespoons minced chipotle peppers in adobo sauce

- 2 tablespoons distilled vinegar

- 1 tablespoon spicy mustard

- 1 tablespoon Worcestershire sauce

Instructions

1. Heat the oil in a saucepan over medium-low heat. Add the garlic and onions and cook for 5 minutes, stirring, being careful not to burn them. Reduce the heat to low. Add the ketchup, molasses, brown sugar, chipotle peppers, vinegar, mustard, and Worcestershire sauce and stir. Allow to simmer for 20 minutes.

Nutrition Facts

Servings: 10

Amount per serving

Calories 95

	% Daily Value*
Total Fat 1.9g	2%
Saturated Fat 0.2g	1%
Cholesterol 2mg	1%
Sodium 432mg	19%
Total Carbohydrate 20.4g	7%
Dietary Fiber 1g	4%
Total Sugars 16.8g	
Protein 0.9g	
Vitamin D 0mcg	0%
Calcium 37mg	3%
Iron 1mg	8%
Potassium 271mg	6%

*The % Daily Value (DV) tells you how much a nutrient in a food serving contributes to a daily diet. 2,000 calorie a day is used for general nutrition advice.

ABOUT THE AUTHOR

I was born and raised in Pittsburgh, Pennsylvania. I earned a Bachelor of Science degree from Virginia State University with a major in Dietetics. My initial interest was to study nursing. However, several conversations with my academic adviser prompted my interest in the study of dietetics. I discovered that this discipline was about more than just food. It was about the science of nutrition and its impact on overall health. Furthermore, I learned of the wide variety of professional organizations where dieticians practiced that included hospitals, public health settings, sports organizations, and outpatient clinics. My new interest converted into a passion for renal health. Upon completing my dietetic internship, I was excited to secure a position on the final rotation in the dialysis unit. Since then, I have been working closely with renal patients to help them through daily struggles. I have learned so much from my patients over the past 15 years, and my passion for renal health continues to grow strong.

Dietary lifestyle is often the source of renal complications. However, I know how difficult it is for patients to adjust to restrictive aspects of the renal diet. There is nothing like the feeling of comfort from down-home cooking! Why should a renal lifestyle change take away this pleasure? It shouldn't and it won't! This is why I created a cookbook to help renal patients continue to enjoy their favorite foods...with a twist! All of the recipes in this resource were modified in my kitchen with a pinch of passion. They have also been tried and tested at recipe showcases where I would seek feedback from my patients who were willing to share their opinion of taste. They have given their stamp of approval! I now have the chance to showcase the recipes with a broader audience in my recipe book. Enjoy!

www.ingramcontent.com/pod-product-compliance
Lightning Source LLC
Chambersburg PA
CBHW060821270326
41931CB00002B/46